Childbirth in Developing Countries

This book is respectfully dedicated to Drs Elton Kessel and Roger P. Bernard for their pioneering work in maternity care monitoring.

Childbirth in Developing Countries

Edited by

**M. Potts, MB, BChir, PhD,
B. Janowitz, PhD, and
J. A. Fortney, PhD**

with the assistance of **E. Jordan**

1983 **MTP PRESS LIMITED**
a member of the KLUWER ACADEMIC PUBLISHERS GROUP
BOSTON / THE HAGUE / DORDRECHT / LANCASTER

Published in the UK and Europe by
MTP Press Limited
Falcon House
Lancaster, England

British Library Cataloguing in Publication Data

Childbirth in developing countries.
   1. Pregnancy—Underdeveloped areas
   2. Childbirth—Underdeveloped area
   I. Potts, M.   II. Janowitz, B.
   III. Fortney, J. A.
   618.2'009172'4   RG551

ISBN 0–85200–493–1

Published in the USA by
MTP Press
A division of Kluwer Boston Inc
190 Old Derby Street
Hingham, MA 02043, USA

Library of Congress Cataloging in Publication Data

Main entry under title:

Childbirth in developing countries.

   Bibliography: p.
   Includes index.
   1. Obstetrics.   2. Childbirth.   3. Underdeveloped areas—Birth
control.   4. Underdeveloped areas—Maternal health services.   I. Potts,
Malcolm.   II. Janowitz, B. (Barbara), 1942–   .   III. Fortney, J. A. (Judith A.),
1938–   . [DNLM: 1. Pregnancy complictions.   2. Cesarean
section.   3. Family planning.   4. Birth
intervals.   5. Contraception.   6. Developing countries.   WQ 240 C536]

RG526.C46 1983   362.1'982'0091723   83–7891
ISBN 0–85200–493–1

Phototypesetting by Georgia Origination, Liverpool
Printed by Butler and Tanner Ltd., Frome and London

Contents

List of Contributors

G. ARAUJO
Sociedade de Assistencia e Maternidade
   Escola Assis Chateaubriand
Fortaleza, Brazil

L. ARAUJO
Sociedade de Assistencia e Maternidade
   Escola Assis Chateaubriand
Fortaleza, Brazil

I. BATAR
Family Planning Center
Dept. of Obstetrics and Gynecology
Medical University
Debrecen, Hungary

I. CHI
Family Health International
Research Triangle Park
North Carolina 27709, USA

D. COVINGTON
Family Health International
Research Triangle Park
North Carolina 27709, USA

A. DIAZ-INFANTE, JR
School of Medicine
Universidad Autonoma de San Luis
   Potosi
San Luis Potosi, Mexico

J. A. FORTNEY
Family Health International
Research Triangle Park
North Carolina 27709, USA

D. E. GUNATILAKE
De Soysa Hospital for Women
Colombo, Sri Lanka

F. HEFNAWI
International Islamic Center for
   Population Studies and Research
Cairo, Egypt

J. E. HIGGINS
Family Health International
Research Triangle Park
North Carolina 27709, USA

B. JANOWITZ
Family Health International
Research Triangle Park
North Carolina 27709, USA

K. I. KENNEDY
Family Health International
Research Triangle Park
North Carolina 27709, USA

L. G. LAMPE
Noi Klinika
Debrecen, Hungary

L. E. LAUFE
University of Texas Health Science
   Center
Department of Obstetrics and
   Gynecology
San Antonio, Texas 78284, USA

J. LEWIS
Family Health International
Research Triangle Park
North Carolina 27709, USA

L. F. MORENO
Hospital Universitario 'Antonio
   Patricio de Alcala'
Cumaná, Venezuela

M. S. NAKAMURA
Pontifical Catholic University of
   Campinas
Campinas, Brazil

D. J. NICHOLS
Family Health International
Research Triangle Park
North Carolina 27709, USA

J. NUNEZ
Family Planning Association of
   Honduras
Tegucigalpa, Honduras

M. POTTS
Family Health International
Research Triangle Park
North Carolina 27709, USA

A. B. SAIFUDDIN
Department of Obstetrics and
   Gynecology
School of Medicine University of
   Indonesia/Dr Cipto Mangunkusumo
   Hospital
Jakarta, Indonesia

S. L. WALLACE
Family Health International
Research Triangle Park
North Carolina 27709, USA

E. W. WHITEHORNE
Family Health International
Research Triangle Park
North Carolina 27709, USA

Acknowledgments

Many investigators in many countries contributed data used in these analyses. While they are too numerous to mention each by name, the editors gratefully acknowledge that without the efforts of these investigators, this book would not have been possible.

Partial support for this work was provided by Family Health International with funds from the US Agency for International Development.

A number of the chapters in this book were previously published or are in press in other publications:

'Childbearing After Age 35: Its Effect on Early Perinatal Outcomes' (Chapter 1) is reproduced from the *Journal of Biosocial Science*, **14,** 69–80, 1982, with permission of the Editor.

'Development of An Index of High-Risk Pregnancy' (Chapter 2) is reproduced from the *American Journal of Obstetrics and Gynecology*, **148**(5), 501–508, July 1, 1982, with permission of the C. V. Mosby Company.

'Cesarean Delivery in Selected Latin American Hospitals' (Chapter 4) is reproduced from *Public Health*, **96,** No. 4, July 1982, with permission of the Editor on behalf of the Society of Community Medicine.

'Deliveries after Cesarean Birth in Two Asian University Hospitals' (Chapter 5) is in press with the *International Journal of Gynaecology & Obstetrics*, and is reproduced by permission of the Editor.

'Child Survivorship and Pregnancy Spacing in Iran' (Chapter 7) is in press with the *Journal of Biosocial Science*, and is reproduced by permission of the Editor.

'Infant and Child Survival and Contraceptive Use in the Closed Pregnancy Interval' (Chapter 8) is in press with *Social Science and Medicine*, and is reproduced by permission of Pergamon Press Ltd.

'Postpartum Sterilization in São Paulo State, Brazil' (Chapter 11) is reproduced from the *Journal of Biosocial Science*, **14**, 179–187, 1982, with permission of the Editor.

'Access to Sterilization in Two Hospitals in Honduras' (Chapter 12) originally appeared in the *Bulletin of the Pan American Health Organization*, 15(3), 226, 1981, and is reproduced with the permission of the authors and the Organization.

Introduction

The need to improve maternal and child health care may be the most important global health need of the remaining years of the twentieth century. It is central to the World Health Organization's (WHO) goal of Health for All by the Year 2000.

The vast majority of births occur in developing countries, where maternity care is often rudimentary. The rates of maternal and infant morbidity and death for these countries are extremely high but much of the morbidity and death is preventable, even with the limited resources available for health care in many parts of the world.

The resources devoted to maternal and child care should be greatly expanded, but even the most hopeful projections will leave a wide gap between human needs and available services. WHO estimates that two billion deliveries in the remaining two decades of this century will not be attended by a trained person. At a minimum, it is probable that two million of these women will die in childbirth.

There were approximately 130 million births in the world in 1980. By the year 2000, this number will reach 163 million. Nearly all this increase in births will occur in developing regions of the world, where 85% of births and 95% of perinatal deaths are expected to occur by the year 2000. In the last two decades of this century, 40 million infants will die in the perinatal period if present rates continue. In all, 250 million or more infant and child deaths will occur[1]. The vast majority of these deaths would be considered preventable by developed-country standards. This tragic loss makes the greatest single contribution to the shorter life expectancy in developing countries.

Although most developing countries have some maternity hospitals in which high-risk deliveries are managed, many are overcrowded and must struggle to provide adequate care with limited financial resources, personnel and facilities. Overall, the resources available for health care in the developing world often remain woefully inadequate (Table 1).

Table 1   Health resources in selected countries, 1980

	Population		
	Per hospital bed	*Per physician*	*Per nurse/midwife*
Ethiopia	3080	69 340	22 320
Sudan	1110	12 680	980
Mengenu	1170	14 810	1620
Bangladesh	5640	15 050	38 560
India	1620	4100	3960
Sri Lanka	330	4010	1300
Indonesia	1560	18 160	4730
Philippines	640	3150	1050
Egypt	470	4630	1870

From: Health Problems and Policies in the Developing Countries. *World Bank Staff Working Paper*, no. 412

An effective solution to the problems of obstetric care can only be developed if the details of those problems are accurately understood. What is the most effective use of limited resources? What are the major causes of death and morbidity? What are the priorities for preventive and curative services? Are some pathologies more common in certain localities and/or groups? How many pregnancies are unplanned? Are realistic and effective family planning services available?

To accelerate development of maternity care in developing countries, health care providers need to know the characteristics of the patients they serve and the risks associated with those characteristics. Collecting information on patients can be an expensive and time-consuming process, even in developed countries. For years, many maternity hospitals and centers in developing countries had no resources to systematically evaluate their services and, therefore, could not determine the most effective means of improving their maternity care services to reduce the number of maternal deaths, still-births and neonatal deaths.

To remedy the shortage of data, a system of maternity care

monitoring (MCM) was developed by Family Health International (FHI), formerly the International Fertility Research Program, Research Triangle Park, NC, USA. MCM was devised to survey broad aspects of maternity care through the routine completion of a simple patient record. The information from the records of all patients in one hospital or center can be analyzed, leading to the identification and quantification of unmet needs in patient management. When the record is used in a representative sample of maternity centers in a country, the resulting information profiles the quality of maternity care in a National Health Service.

DEVELOPMENT OF MATERNITY CARE MONITORING

In 1974 Dr Hamid Rushwan of Khartoum in the Sudan suggested that FHI develop a form to collect information on deliveries. Dr Rushwan had participated in FHI's clinical trials and was particularly pleased with the rapid feedback, in the form of standardized computer analysis tables, that he received. Similar feedback on obstetric cases would, he pointed out, not only facilitate the writing of annual reports, but would also have an important potential for the improvement of patient care. Although his hospital collected information on deliveries, any analysis required tedious hand tabulation and as a consequence little analysis was done.

Following Dr Rushwan's suggestion, FHI developed a local Maternity Record to be completed for each woman admitted to a maternity center for delivery. This Record was developed through a trial-and-error process that lasted more than 2 years. The first trial was done in Khartoum with Dr Rushwan at the request of the Sudanese Fertility Control Association. FHI also received much encouragement from Dr Hubert de Watteville, then Secretary General of the International Federation of Gynaecology and Obstetrics (FIGO), and a pretest was conducted in approximately 30 maternity centers in 1976 as a co-operative effort between FHI and FIGO. When early findings showed the potential of this approach, the pretest was expanded. Since that time, FIGO has supported the concept of maternity care monitoring and, in 1978, its Executive Board, under Dr de Watteville's successor, Dr John Tomkinson, recommended the Maternity Record to all national societies of gynecology and obstetrics. Among the many FHI staff who worked on MCM, founder Dr Elton Kessel took a special interest and Dr Roger Bernard put a great deal of energy into the early data analysis.

The Division of Family Health of the WHO reviewed the preliminary analyses and data collection instruments in late 1977. They encouraged both FIGO and FHI to broaden the testing at the institutional level and urged a move toward use in peripheral centers in non-urban areas, where the need for this type of monitoring system is the greatest.

The first national experience with the Maternity Record, a stratified random sample of 40 urban hospitals, occurred in Colombia. This national profile of maternity care management was used by the Ministry of Health to identify areas in the Colombian maternity care system needing improvement.

Since its beginnings, the Maternity Record (reproduced on pages xix–xxi) has received international recognition as an interdisciplinary data source, and as an invaluable tool for monitoring events in maternity centers. When analyzed, the data collected by the Record are useful to clinicians, program administrators, health planners and researchers as a comprehensive summary of events in the maternity ward.

The stated objectives of the Maternity Record are:

(1) To provide information on the reproductive histories of women to identify groups at increased risk of complications.
(2) To provide information on selected antenatal conditions that may contribute to identifying factors affecting pregnancy outcome and maternal health.
(3) To provide information on the management and outcome of deliveries that may help identify specific management techniques to improve pregnancy outcome.
(4) To provide information on family size expectations and contraceptive behavior to determine whether hospitals are meeting the family planning needs of their patients.
(5) To provide a source of current information for developing instructional materials to improve standards of teaching and training in health.

The data referred to throughout this book were collected on the single-sheet Record. The Record is completed during hospital admission for each woman who is admitted to and who subsequently delivers at the hospital, regardless of delivery outcome. Thus, data include all births occurring at the center during the reporting period. Health personnel in participating institutions complete the Records using definitions and criteria provided in the Maternity Record Instruction Manual and send the Records to FHI for analysis. FHI sends the participating institutions computerized standard analysis tables at specified intervals.

Overall, MCM has much to contribute to the optimum use of the limited resources available for maternal and infant care. Although the Maternity Record was designed to meet developing world needs, it has proven useful in developed countries. By October 1982, the MCM system has accumulated histories of over 450 000 deliveries occurring at more than 150 maternity centers in 39 developing and developed countries.

PLAN OF THE BOOK

The Maternity Record has proved to be useful not only as a monitoring tool but also in providing information on a variety of topics of general interest to obstetricians, health administrators and social scientists. These topics include management of high-risk pregnancies and referral patterns among institutions offering different levels of care, determinants and implications of cesarean delivery in different types of hospitals, postpartum contraception and breast-feeding, maternal and perinatal mortality, and the consequences of early and late childbearing. Over the past several years, FHI staff have worked with collaborating investigators in preparing a large number of papers on several of these topics. Often the contributors specifically request the data analysis. On other occasions, the staff at FHI suggested that certain problems be examined. The papers in this book are a compilation of some of the combined efforts of FHI staff and collaborating investigators.

The first section of the book consists of three chapters on high-risk pregnancy. Fertility in developing countries is characterized by childbearing at the extreme ages of the reproductive span. The first chapter refers to childbearing among women 35 and older, and finds that in the two developing country hospitals, the babies born to older women are more likely to die before their mothers are discharged from the hospital, and that they are also more likely to have lower Apgar scores. In the one developed country hospital, however, this was not the case.

These mothers were at lower risk than their counterparts in developing countries for a variety of other reasons.

The second chapter discusses the construction of risk indices. Although risk indices are necessary to any referral system, the shortcomings are inherent, and too great demands should not be made of them.

The third chapter concerns questions relating to the allocation of resources for obstetric care in settings in which traditional birth attendants (TBAs) play a significant role. In the developing world, shortages of doctors, especially in rural areas, necessitate that other health workers provide obstetric care. Throughout Third World countries, a significant percentage of deliveries occur at home and are often assisted by traditional birth attendants. Upgrading the skills of TBAs and incorporating them into the health care network can significantly improve maternal and child health. The chapter discusses an innovative TBA training program in Northeast Brazil, which includes the setting up of obstetric units staffed by TBAs and the referral of high-risk cases to a well-staffed and well-equipped hospital in a nearby city.

In the United States, issues relating to cesarean delivery have played an important role in obstetric research. Two questions of major concern are (1) the choice of delivery for infants in the breech presentation and (2) the feasibility of allowing a trial of labor for women with a previous cesarean delivery. Both these questions are addressed in the chapters in the second section of this book. There are also pronounced geographical differences in the propensity to deliver abdominally that go beyond patient characteristics and hospital resources.

The first chapter of this section (Chapter 4) addresses this issue in the context of selected hospitals in Latin America. Because of the large size of the data set, factors associated with rare events can be studied. Only 3–4% of all babies are in the breech position, but analysis focusing on the relative merits of cesarean over vaginal delivery requires a large data set if type of breech presentation, birth weight, etc. are to be controlled. More than 11 000 breech births were available for analysis.

In the United States, although a few researchers have suggested that it is an acceptable practice to allow selected patients with a previous cesarean a trial of labor, over 99% of infants born to women with a previous cesarean delivery are delivered abdominally. In hospitals in developing countries, many women with a previous cesarean delivery have a subsequent vaginal delivery. Thus, data from hospitals in developing countries can be useful in understanding the ramifications of allowing US women a trial of labor.

While some investigators have argued that the rate of cesarean delivery in the United States is too high, the rate in several Brazilian hospitals (and probably in the country as a whole) is much higher, but rates in hospitals in other Latin American countries are much lower than in the United States. This chapter examines the reasons for this diversity and considers the benefits of a reduction in the rate of cesarean delivery in hospitals with the highest rates.

The determinants and consequences of the interval between pregnancies is discussed in the three chapters (7–9) in the third section. The data used were collected at what used to be known as the Queen Farah Maternity Hospital in Tehran, Iran.

While there is a growing literature on the determinants of the length of the pregnancy interval, much of the available data used suffers from a number of drawbacks – small sample size and recall of long-past events. Maternity Record data are free of these limitations and, therefore, provide a unique opportunity to study determinants of pregnancy intervals by cross-classifying women according to the outcome of their last pregnancy, breast-feeding status of that child if born alive and contraceptive use of the interval preceding the current pregnancy.

One of the most important determinants of the length of the pregnancy interval is, of course, whether the mother practiced contraception at any time in the interval. The second chapter (Chapter 8) analyzes the determinants of contraceptive status, and finds that the outcome of the previous pregnancy is an important indicator of whether or not the woman used contraception. Therefore, where poor pregnancy outcome is common, public health programs that improve survival status would also increase the use of family planning.

The last chapter (Chapter 9) discusses the consequences of spacing. While this, too, has been a widely researched topic, this analysis is unique in that the outcome of the previous pregnancy is controlled, and the complex interrelationship between birth interval and maternal age and parity is examined.

For many women, the stimulus to adopt contraception is the birth of a child and if the pregnancy was unwanted, this birth may be the stimulus to choose sterilization. The chapters in the final section (10–12) focus on postpartum plans for contraception and the factors affecting the provision of surgical sterilization at hospitals in two different countries.

While the Maternity Record provides data on planned rather than actual contraception (except in the case of postpartum sterilization), these data are useful in understanding the factors that motivate women to plan to adopt or continue the use of contraception. The first chapter (Chapter 10) in this group examines postpartum contraceptive plans among women delivering at Al Galaa Maternity Hospital in Cairo, Egypt. This chapter establishes the links between the survival status of a woman's previous pregnancies (especially her most recent), her desire for additional children and her subsequent plans for contraception.

The final two chapters (11 and 12) examine the provision of surgical sterilization in hospitals in Brazil and Honduras. Results show that both the physical capability of the hospital in providing services and the policies followed by the hospital in making services available can affect access to postpartum sterilization. In Honduras, crowded operating rooms prevent almost all women with vaginal deliveries from having a tubal ligation, as the hospitals generally restrict sterilization to women with cesarean deliveries (who often have medical indications for sterilization). In the Brazilian hospitals, private patients are more likely to have cesarean deliveries and, therefore, tubal ligations than are women whose care is funded through the public sector. In this case, it is the institutional arrangements surrounding the system of payment that make it difficult for poor women to undergo a postpartum sterilization.

Reference

1 Gwatkin, D. R. (1980). How many die? A set of demographic estimates of the annual number of infant and child deaths in the world. *Am. J. Public Health*, 70, 1286

INTERNATIONAL FERTILITY RESEARCH PROGRAM
MATERNITY RECORD

PATIENT IDENTIFICATION: 1. Hospital or clinic no. _____

2. Admission date _____ _____ _____
   day   month   year

3. Patient's name _____   _____   _____   _____
                    family   first   maiden   Husband's name

4. Address _____

STUDY IDENTIFICATION

5. Center name _____ and number: | | | | 1-3

6. Study number: | 9 | 0 | 3 | 4-6

7. Patient order number: | | | | | | 7-11

8. Delivery date: | | | | | | | 12-17
   day   month   year

9. Registration status: 0) not booked 1) booked, patient's choice 2) referred by physician 3) referred by midwife 4) emergency, 8) other _____ | | 18

PATIENT CHARACTERISTICS

10. Residence: 1) urban 2) rural 3) urban slum 4) rural slum | | 19

11. Patient's status: 1) private 2) not private 8) other | | 20

12. Patient's age: *(completed years)* | | | | 21-22

13. Patient's education: *(school year completed)* 0) 0 1) 1-2 2) 3-4 3) 5-6 4) 7-8 5) 9-10 6) 11-12 7) 13-14 8) 15+ | | 23

14. Marital status: 1) never married 2) currently married 3) divorced 4) separated 5) widowed 6) consensual union 8) other | | | | 24

15. Age at first marriage/union: *(completed years)* | | | | 25-26

36. Anesthetic administered: 0) none or psychoprophylaxis only 1) analgesic, systemic or inhalation 2) local 3) paracervical/pudendal 4) spinal/epidural 5) general 6) 1 and 2 or 1 and 3 7) other combination 8) other _____ | | 52

37. Episiotomy: 0) none 1) midline 2) midline, with extension 3) midline, with hematoma 4) mediolateral 5) mediolateral, with extension 6) mediolateral, with hematoma 8) other | | 53

38. Type of delivery: 0) spontaneous 1) outlet forceps 2) vacuum extractor 3) mid- or high forceps 4) manual rotation 5) breech extraction 6) cesarean section 7) destructive procedure 8) other _____ | | 54

39. Primary injury during labor and/or delivery: 0) none 1) vulva 2) vagina 3) perineum 4) cervix 5) uterus 6) rectum 7) bladder 8) other _____ | | 55

40. Primary complication of labor and/or delivery: 0) none 1) prolonged/obstructed labor 2) placenta previa 3) placenta abruptio 4) hypotonic uterine contractions 5) hypertonic uterine contractions 6) hemorrhage 7) retained products 8) other _____ | | 56

41. Secondary complication of labor and/or delivery: 0) none 1) prolonged labor 2) cord prolapse 4) hypotonic uterine contractions 5) hypertonic uterine contractions 6) hemorrhage 7) retained products 8) other _____ | | 57

OBSTETRIC HISTORY (not including this pregnancy)

16. Total live births: ⬜⬜ `27–28`

17. Children now living:
        number of males ⬜ `29`
    (8 or more = 8)
        number of females ⬜ `30`

18. Duration of breast-feeding of last live birth:
(in months) 0) did not breast-feed 1) <3 2) <6
3) <9 4) <12 5) <15 6) <18 7) <21 8) ≥21 ⬜ `31`

19. Number of stillbirths: *(8 or more = 8)* ⬜ `32`

20. Number of infant deaths: *(less than 12 completed months; 8 or more = 8)* ⬜ `33`

21. Number of spontaneous abortions: *(8 or more = 8)* ⬜ `34`

22. Number of induced abortions: *(8 or more = 8)* ⬜ `35`

23. Outcome of last pregnancy: 0) not previously pregnant 1) live birth, full term, still living 2) live birth, full term, deceased 3) live birth, premature, still living 4) live birth, premature, deceased 5) stillbirth 6) induced abortion 7) spontaneous abortion 8) other ⬜ `36`

24. Number of months since last pregnancy ended: *(98 or more = 98)* ⬜⬜ `37–38`

25. Contraceptive method mainly used before conception: 0) none 1) IUD 2) orals/injectables 3) female sterilization 4) male sterilization 5) condom 6) withdrawal/rhythm 7) foam/diaphragm/jelly 8) other _____ ⬜ `39`

MEDICAL DATA

26. Number of antenatal visits: *(8 or more = 8)* ⬜ `40`

27. Primary antenatal condition: *(see code list)* ⬜⬜ `41–42`

42. Duration of labor: *(in completed hours)* 0) none 1) <2 2) 2-6 3) 7-12 4) 13-18 5) 19-24 6) 25-48 7) over 48 ⬜ `58`

43. Attendant at delivery: 0) none 1) nurse 2) qualified midwife 3) student nurse/midwife 4) paramedic 5) medical student 6) general physician 7) OB/GYN physician 8) other ⬜ `59`

44. Birth weight: *(gm: 9988 or more = 9988)* ⬜⬜⬜ `60–62`

45. Sex of infant(s) born   number of males ⬜ `63`
at this delivery: *(write number of each)*
           number of females ⬜ `64`

46. Apgar score: 9) not done   at 1 minute ⬜ `65`
        (8 or more = 8)
           at 5 minutes ⬜ `66`

For Items 47-48, use the following codes: 0) normal or stillbirth with no apparent pathology 1) fetal distress during labor 2) minor malformation 3) major malformation 4) respiratory distress syndrome 5) isoimmunization 6) neonatal sepsis 7) trauma 8) other *(for codes 2, 3, 7 and 8, specify)*

47. Primary fetal/neonatal condition, specify _____ ⬜ `67`

48. Secondary fetal/neonatal condition, specify _____ ⬜ `68`

49. Death of fetus/newborn: 0) none 1) antepartum, one 2) antepartum, two or more 3) intrapartum, one 4) intrapartum two or more 5) postpartum, one 6) postpartum, two or more 7) combination 8) other ⬜ `69`

50. Primary puerperal condition: 0) normal 1) fever requiring treatment 2) bleeding requiring treatment 3) urinary tract infection 4) mastitis 5) phlebitis 6) dehiscence 7) death *(complete Death Report)* 8) other _____ ⬜ `70`

28. Hospitalization required during this pregnancy: 0) no 1) yes, for condition indicated in Item 27 2) yes, for condition other than the one indicated in Item 27, specify condition _____

☐ 43

29. Tobacco smoking during pregnancy: 0) none **During part of pregnancy** *(cigarettes/day)*: 1) 1-10 2) 11-20 3) 21 or more **Throughout pregnancy** *(cigarettes/day)*: 4) 1-10 5) 11-20 6) 21 or more 8) cigars, pipes, etc

☐☐ 44 45

30. Number of previous cesarean sections:

☐ 46-47

31. Estimated duration of pregnancy: *(menstrual age in completed weeks)*

☐ 48

32. Hemoglobin at admission for delivery (to nearest gm): 1) ≤5 gm 2) 6 gm 3) 7 gm 4) 8 gm 5) 9 gm 6) 10 gm 7) 11 gm 8) ≥12 gm 9) not done

☐ 49

33. Rupture of membranes: **Spontaneous:** 1) <24 hrs before delivery 2) ≥24 hrs before delivery **Artificial:** 3) <24 hours before delivery 4) ≥24 hrs before delivery 5) during cesarean section

☐ 50

34. Type of labor: 0) no labor 1) spontaneous 2) spontaneous, augmented with artificial rupture of membranes (ARM) 3) spontaneous, augmented with drugs 4) spontaneous, augmented with ARM and drugs 5) induced, with ARM 6) induced, with drugs 7) induced, with ARM and drugs 8) other

For multiple births, code information for the most difficult delivery in Items 35, 38, 44, 46, 47 and 48 and complete a separate Multiple Birth Record for each infant.

35. Type of presentation during labor: 0) vertex, occiput anterior 1) vertex, occiput transverse or posterior 2) frank breech 3) footling breech 4) complete breech 5) brow/face 6) transverse lie 7) compound 8) other

☐ 51

---

51. Maternal blood transfusion during hospitalization: 0) none 1) yes, before delivery 2) yes, during delivery 3) yes, after delivery 4) 1 and 2 5) 1 and 3 6) 2 and 3 7) 1, 2 and 3

☐ 71

52. Number of nights hospitalized this admission before delivery: *(8 or more = 8)*

☐ 72

SPECIAL STUDIES

53. ☐☐☐ 73 74 75

54. _____

55. _____

Complete these items at time of discharge:

56. Number of nights hospitalized this admission after delivery: *(8 or more = 8)*

☐ 76

57. Female sterilization: 0) none 1) before this delivery 2) at cesarean section 3) immediately after delivery 4) same day 5) 1-2 days later 6) 3-4 days later 7) 5-9 days later 8) 10 or more days later

☐☐ 77 78

58. Number of additional children wanted: *(8 or more = 8)*

59. Contraceptive method planned or provided: 0) none 1) IUD 2) orals/injectables 3) female sterilization 4) male sterilization 5) condom 6) withdrawal/rhythm 7) foam/diaphragm/jelly 8) other _____

☐ 79   ☐ **1** 80

Recorder's name

PLEASE AIRMAIL TO: *International Fertility Research Program, Research Triangle Park, North Carolina 27709 USA*

MAT 001 12/78

Section I:
HIGH-RISK PREGNANCY

1

Childbearing after age 35: its effect on early perinatal outcomes

J. A. FORTNEY, J. E. HIGGINS, A. DIAZ-INFANTE, Jr,
F. HEFNAWI, L. G. LAMPE and I. BATAR

In many developing countries many births are to women 35 years or older. The risk of adverse maternal and fetal outcome is greater with increasing age, and so is the risk of certain congenital malformations. These risks have been well summarized by Nortman[10].

In a relatively large collaborative study (1835 gravidas aged 35 and over), Israel and Deutschberger[5] found there was a significant increase with age in stillbirth rates, but that older women had *lower* rates of neonatal deaths. This can presumably be attributed to the fact that neonatal deaths are affected by environmental as well as congenital factors. Other authors have concluded that there is a real (i.e. physiological) relationship between maternal age and stillbirths; however, Resseguie[11] has made a plausible argument that, in the United States at least, this relationship is an artifact of analysis rather than a genuine increase in risk. 'When births to mothers . . . are subdivided according to the amount of education completed by the mother, the association between stillbirth rate and maternal age in each educational group differs substantially from the others.' Baird, on the other hand, found that the influence of age on perinatal mortality was not affected when social class was controlled[1].

The increased incidence of depressed Apgar scores (a score of <7 representing neonatal morbidity) has been commented upon by many authors[2,8], as has the increased incidence of low-birth-weight infants[2,6,9]. However, some authors have found that the difference in birth weight was not statistically significant for primigravidas[8].

Although the relative risk for older women is high compared with gravidas in the low-risk childbearing years (20–34), the absolute risk can be quite low depending on the management of the pregnancy. Obstetricians in developed countries are anticipating an increase in the number of elderly primigravidas and low-parity gravidas as delayed childbearing becomes more common. Daniels and Weingarten[3] have satisfactorily summarized the risks of postponed childbearing in the United States.

Although late childbearing in developed countries often involves low parity women, in developing countries it is more likely to involve grandmultiparas (women with four or more previous live births). This paper, therefore, compares the outcome of deliveries to women 35 or older with women in the low-risk ages (20–34) in three very different cultural settings, Mexico, Egypt and Hungary. Data from three hospitals – one in each country – are analyzed. Since these are hospital deliveries, the findings cannot be generalized to these countries as a whole, the more so since all three of these hospitals are urban teaching and referral centers. Because of this, it is probable that patients admitted are not representative of women delivering in the catchment area; in particular they may be more likely to have a higher rate of complications, and are, perhaps, more likely to be older. Nevertheless, the percentage of births to older women is not greater in these hospitals than in the country as a whole, as Table 1 shows.

The number of cases and the range of dates analyzed in this study are as follows:

Mexico	5379 cases	7 March '77 to 6 April '80
Egypt	7355 cases	1 March '77 to 1 April '80
Hungary	11 278 cases	1 Jan '77 to 5 Aug '80

The three hospitals were selected because of the large number of older women delivering there; although the number in the Hungarian hospital is much smaller than in the other two hospitals (see Table 1), it is the only hospital from a developed country sending data to FHI for which there are sufficient cases for analysis.

Compared with the national data of 3–5 years earlier (Table 1), the FHI data for Mexico show a greater percentage of the older women to be grandmultiparas and a smaller percentage (3·2% compared with 9·5%) to be primiparas. For Egypt, there is a greater similarity in the percentage who are primiparas (3·1% in the FHI data compared with

3·4% in the national data), but the FHI data show a percentage of
patients of parity 10 or higher that is more than twice the rate in the
earlier national data. The FHI data for Hungary show a larger percentage of primiparas (21·2% compared with 11·4% in the national
data) and a correspondingly smaller percentage of grandmultiparas
(10·7% compared with 29·9% in the national data).

It is apparent that older women who deliver tend to have characteristics in addition to their age that contribute to their risk status. Most
obviously, they tend to be of high parity; the last line of Table 1 shows
the percentage of obstetric patients aged 35 or older with at least ten
previous live births, and Table 2 shows the mean parity for each of

Table 1   Distribution of births by age of mother in Mexico, Egypt and Hungary:
selected characteristics of births to mothers over 35 years

	Mexico		Egypt		Hungary	
	UN* 1973	FHI† 1977–80	UN* 1973	FHI† 1977–79	UN* 1974	FHI† 1977–80
Total no. of births	2 572 287	7085	1 259 004	8379	186 288	12 581
% in each age group‡						
< 20	12·4	22·8	3·5	8·9	15·1	9·1
20–24	25·2	27·5	21·1	30·7	42·4	42·3
25–29	23·4	18·7	27·6	27·9	26·2	31·7
30–34	16·5	13·4	21·2	17·3	11·7	12·1
35–39	12·7	11·6	15·8	11·6	3.7	3.6
40+	8·1	6·0	8·7	3·6	0·9	1·1
35+	20·8	17·6	24·5	15·1	4·6	4·7
No. of births to women 35+	535 490	1247	308 823	1269	8577	592
% of births to women 35+						
First births	9·5	3·2	3·4	3·1	11·4	21·2
5th and higher order	66·7	82·6	62·2	65·9	29·9	10·7
10th and higher order	20·2	34·5	3·1	7·6	5·9	2·1

* National data. Source: *Demographic Yearbook, 1975*, United Nations
† Family Health International data
‡ May not equal 100% because some mothers are of unknown age

three age groups in the three hospitals. In the Mexican hospital, in particular, the oldest parturients tend to be of very high parity (9·2 live births). In the Hungarian hospital, as might be expected, a much smaller percentage are of very high parity, and the mean parity of the women over 40 is 2·8 live births. As well as the additional risk from high parity, older obstetric patients are less likely to seek antenatal care, and are likely to have less education than younger patients – both factors that are associated with increased obstetric risk. Table 2 shows the distribution of each of these variables with respect to age for the three hospitals.

Thus it is necessary to control for these additional characteristics in examining the relationship between maternal age and the fetal outcome variables. To this end, the Mantel–Haenszel[7] procedure was used to test the statistical significance, via a chi-square test statistic, of the relationship after controlling for the additional factors. Use of the Mantel–Haenszel statistic in the case of no controls yields results almost identical to the commonly used Pearson chi-square statistic when the sample size is large. Throughout this paper, the 0·05 level of statistical significance is used, and the word significance, where used in the remainder of this paper, refers to statistical significance.

Table 2 Selected maternal characteristics by age of mother: Mexico, Egypt and Hungary

Characteristic/age group	Mexico	Egypt	Hungary
Mean years of schooling			
20–34	4·4	3·4	11·2
35–39	2·4	1·6	10·6
40+	1·9	1·1	8·1
Mean parity			
20–34	2·2	1·6	0·7
35–39	7·4	5·2	1·8
40+	9·2	6·7	2·8
Mean no. of antenatal visits			
20–34	1·2	1·0	7·4
35–39	1·1	1·0	7·1
40+	1·0	1·1	6·4
% with no antenatal care			
20–34	64·2	66·9	1·0
35–39	66·9	67·3	1·6
40+	69·1	66·1	4·6

Three outcome variables were examined: (1) depressed Apgar score, (2) low birth weight and (3) survival. For each data set, the association between age and each outcome variable is tested both without controlling for other factors and with control for factors one at a time.

DEPRESSED APGAR SCORE

An Apgar score of < 7 at 5 minutes is generally regarded as indicating neonatal morbidity. As shown in the first two rows of Table 3, older women in the Mexican and Egyptian hospitals have a significantly larger percentage of babies with a depressed Apgar score when other factors are not controlled. In the Mexican hospital, 2·6% of the live-born babies of the younger mothers had a depressed Apgar score at 5 minutes, compared with 5·1% of the older mothers. In the Egyptian hospital, the comparable percentages were 2·4 and 3·8. In the Hungarian hospital, however, there was no difference, 0·6% of the infants of both groups of mothers had a low Apgar score.

In the Mexican hospital, the association between age and Apgar score remains significant when each of the covariables is controlled. For the levels of all the covariables except parity, the older women have a larger percentage of babies with a depressed Apgar score. Evidence of such an association is less consistent in the Egyptian hospital data where residence is the only covariable having both a higher percentage of depressed Apgar scores in the older age group for each type of residence and a significant Mantel–Haenszel test statistic. Although the test statistics are significant when controlling for either education or smoking, the intra-level evidence is not consistent (e.g. older non-smokers show a higher percentage of depressed Apgar scores while older smokers do not). Finally, the Hungarian hospital data produce no significant tests of association when each of the covariables is controlled.

LOW BIRTH WEIGHT

Table 4 shows the percentage of infants weighing less than 2500 g at birth for each of the three hospitals, as well as for the levels of the several related variables. In each of the three hospitals, a higher percentage of older mothers had low-birth-weight babies; the difference

Table 3 Percentage of infants with Apgar scores of less than seven at 5 minutes, by age and other selected characteristics: Mexico, Egypt and Hungary

Type of comparison	Characteristic	Mexico 20–34 (4162)†	Mexico 35+ (1217)	Egypt 20–34 (6134)	Egypt 35+ (1221)	Hungary 20–34 (10697)	Hungary 35+ (581)
Age with	Total	2·6	5·1	2·4	3·8	0·6	0·6
Apgar	M–H χ^2‡		16·5*		6·5*		0·1
Age with	Parity						
Apgar	0	3·2	3·0	2·4	3·7	0·6	0·0
controlling	1–3	2·3	3·4	2·0	4·1	0·6	0·6
for	4+	2·7	5·5	3·4	3·7	0·0	1·4
parity	M–H χ^2		9·7*		1·6		0·1
Age with Apgar	Antenatal visits						
controlling	0	2·7	6·0	2·4	4·1	1·9	0·0
for	1–4	2·7	3·4	2·4	2·1	0·8	3·3
antenatal	5+	1·5	3·4	2·1	6·8	0·6	0·4
visits	M–H χ^2		16·0*		1·6		0·1
Age with	Education (years)						
Apgar	0	4·3	6·0	2·6	4·3	0·0	0·0
controlling	1–6	2·2	4·4	2·1	2·6	0·8	0·0
for	7+	2·5	8·3	2·4	2·1	0·6	0·7
education	M–H χ^2		10·0*		5·0*		0·1
Age with	Residence						
Apgar	Urban	1·8	4·6	2·4	3·2	0·5	0·0
controlling	Rural	3·4	5·7	3·5	4·8	0·9	2·0
for	Slum	3·5	4·5	1·6	4·3		
residence	M–H χ^2		13·0*		6·2*		0·1
Age with Apgar	Smoking						
controlling	No	2·5	5·1	1·8	3·3	0·6	0·5
for	Yes	2·9	5·6	2·1	0·0	0·0	2·3
smoking	M–H χ^2		16·9*		5·9*		0·2

† n in parentheses
‡ Mantel–Haenszel
* Significant at $\alpha=0·05$, Pr $(1 \, df\chi^2 \langle 3·84) = 0·05$

was small in Mexico and Egypt and not statistically significant. Only in Hungary was the difference of a magnitude (16·0% compared with 11·2%) to achieve statistical significance.

When other variables are controlled, the same pattern remains. None of the Mantel–Haenszel statistics, when the covariables are controlled singly, achieves significance in either the Mexican or Egyptian data sets. For the Hungarian data, however, there is a

Table 4 Percentage of infants weighing less than 2500 g by age and by other selected characteristics: Mexico, Egypt and Hungary

		Age (years)					
		Mexico		Egypt		Hungary	
Type of comparison	Characteristic	20–34 (4162)†	35+ (1217)	20–34 (6134)	35+ (1221)	20–34 (10 697)	35+ (581)
Age with	Total	11·9	12·3	7·2	7·4	11·2	16·0
birthweight	M–H x^2‡	0·1		0·1		12·4*	
Age with	Parity						
birthweight	0	15·0	5·1	6·4	5·9	11·3	20·2
controlling	1–3	11·0	14·2	7·3	6·7	11·0	12·8
for	4+	10·8	12·2	8·7	7·6	20·2	21·1
parity	M–H x^2	0·8		0·9		5·5*	
Age with							
birthweight	Antenatal visits						
controlling	0	12·2	13·2	6·6	7·6	35·8	30·8
for	1–4	11·7	11·6	8·4	7·4	35·6	38·0
antenatal	5+	11·3	7·1	8·8	5·4	9·9	13·5
visits	M–H x^2	1·5		<0·1		5·8*	
Age with	Education (years)						
birthweight	0	13·7	12·8	7·1	7·1	21·2	33·3
controlling	1–6	11·7	12·0	7·3	8·3	24·1	20·0
for	7+	10·7	11·1	7·4	8·5	11·0	14·8
education	M–H x^2	0·1		<0·1		4·7*	
Age with	Residence						
birthweight	Urban	11·5	10·8	7·6	7·1	10·4	14·7
controlling	Rural	12·2	14·8	5·8	8·2	14·4	18·8
for	Slum	13·0	6·0	7·5	7·5	—	—
residence	M–H x^2	<0·1		<0·1		9·8*	
Age with							
birthweight	Smoking						
controlling	No	12·0	12·6	7·7	7·7	9·7	15·0
for	Yes	12·0	7·2	6·7	5·3	22·2	27·9
smoking	M–H x^2	<0·1		<0·1		13·7*	

† n in parentheses
‡ Mantel–Haenszel
* Significant at $\alpha = 0\cdot05$, Pr (1 dfx^2 ⟨3·84⟩ = 0·05

significant increase in the percentage of low-birth-weight babies for older women after controlling in turn for each of the covariables. Further, the levels of parity, residence and smoking are consistent in the intra-level percentages of low birth weight. By applying the categorical data analysis methods of Grizzle, Starmer and Koch[4], the relative importance of age, parity, antenatal visits, education, residence and smoking was established for the Hungarian data. Smoking offered by far the most explanatory information regarding the variability of birth weight, while age had a less significant effect than either antenatal visits, education or parity.

SURVIVAL

The survival measure used here (the percentage of infants surviving until the mother's discharge from the hospital) does not necessarily reflect perinatal survival since it depends on the duration of hospitalization. Nevertheless, it is the only available approximation of perinatal survival in the data. Although we cannot precisely estimate perinatal survival, we can still test differences in infant survival between the two age groups by controlling, via the Mantel–Haenszel procedure, for the duration of mother's hospital stay after delivery. The survival percentages in Tables 5 and 6 are not adjusted for duration of mother's hospital stay after delivery, but the test statistics are.

In each of the three hospitals, the percentage of normal-weight babies (at least 2500 g) still alive when the mother was discharged from the hospital decreased with maternal age (Table 5). In Mexico, 96·1% of the infants of the younger mothers survived until discharge, compared with 90·7% of the infants of the older mothers, a significant difference. In Egypt, the comparable percentages are 94·9 and 87·7 (significant difference); while in Hungary there was virtually no difference in the survival until discharge of the two groups of infants (comparable percentages are 98·9 and 98·4).

Because of the interrelationship between maternal age, infant survival and several other factors, Table 5 shows the relationship between maternal age and infant survival with each of the other factors controlled. When the covariables are controlled one at a time, all of the Mantel–Haenszel statistics are significant for the Mexican and Egyptian data, but none reach significance in the Hungarian data. Further, with the exception of education in Mexico and smoking in Egypt, all levels of the covariables show a decline in the percentage of the survival measure in the older mothers.

Among the low-birth-weight infants (shown in Table 6), the survival percentages are, of course, much lower than for the normal-birth-weight infants. As with the normal-birth-weight infants, the survival percentages are significantly less among the older women in Mexico and Egypt but not in Hungary. Likewise, the pattern of differences extends to the levels of the covariates. For the Mexican and Egyptian data, the Mantel–Haenszel statistics are all significant when controlling for the covariables individually; none are significant in the Hungarian data. Furthermore, except for two levels with small cell

Table 5 Percentage of infants weighing 2500 g or more who survive until the mother's discharge from the hospital, by age and other selected characteristics: Mexico, Egypt and Hungary

Type of comparison	Characteristic	Age (years)					
		Mexico		Egypt		Hungary	
		20–34 (3665)†	35+ (1067)	20–34 (5690)	35+ (1131)	20–34 (9497)	35+ (488)
Age with survival	Total	96·1	90·7	94·9	87·8	98·9	98·4
Age with	M–H χ^2‡	45·6*		65·7*		0·5	
survival	Parity						
Age with survival	0	96·7	89·2	96·0	87·5	99·0	100.0
controlling	1–3	96·6	95·6	95·3	90·5	99·0	97·8
for	4+	94·9	90·3	91·8	87·3	96·1	98·6
parity	M–H χ^2	17·7*		19·8*		0·1	
Age with survival	Antenatal visits						
controlling	0	95·3	89·5	94·7	86·9	86·9	77·8
for	1–4	97·8	92·6	95·6	89·2	87·9	96·8
antenatal	5+	96·8	95·6	95·3	90·9	99·4	98·9
visits	M–H χ^2	45·6*		82·9*		<0·1	
Age with	Education (years)						
survival	0	93·3	90·5	93·5	88·1	96·2	90·0
controlling	1–6	96·4	90·5	96·3	85·7	98·4	100·0
for	7+	98·5	100·0	96·7	92·6	98·9	98·3
education	M–H χ^2	41·6*		72·0*		<0·1	
Age with	Residence						
survival	Urban	98·1	93·5	95·0	86·6	99·1	99·4
controlling	Rural	94·1	88·2	93·8	89·7	98·3	96·2
for	Slum	93·9	93·0	95·5	88·7	—	—
residence	M–H χ^2	33·7		82·2*		0·1	
Age with survival	Smoking						
controlling	No	96·0	91·0	94·9	87·1	98·9	98·2
for	Yes	97·2	89·6	92·9	94·4	98·4	97·7
smoking	M–H χ^2	42·6*		66·2		0·5	

† n in parentheses
‡ Mantel–Haenszel
* Significant at $\alpha = 0·05$, Pr (1 df $\chi^2 \langle 3·84 \rangle = 0·05$

sizes, the survival percentages are consistently smaller among the older women when the covariable levels are considered.

To summarize, although it is generally true that factors influencing perinatal mortality do so by operating through the mechanism of birth weight, this does not appear to be the case where advanced maternal

Table 6   Percentage of infants weighing less than 2500 g who survive until the mother's discharge from the hospital, by age and other selected characteristics: Mexico, Egypt and Hungary

		Age (years)					
		Mexico		Egypt		Hungary	
Type of comparison	Characteristic	20–34 (497)†	35+ (150)	20–34 (443)	35+ (90)	20–34 (1200)	35+ (93)
Age with	Total	76·3	58·0	64·9	44·4	82·0	84·9
survival	M–H χ^2‡	13·7*		10·2*		0·8	
Age with	Parity						
survival	0	84·7	100·0	76·5	50·0	81·1	88·0
controlling	1–3	73·7	53·3	56·9	50·0	83·2	80·4
for	4+	71·0	57·4	63·9	43·2	73·1	89·5
parity	M–H χ^2	5·6*		6·1*		0·6*	
Age with	Antenatal visits						
survival							
controlling	0	72·9	55·0	64·2	45·2	44·1	50·0
for	1–4	79·5	64·7	71·2	43·5	68·1	84·2
antenatal	5+	90·0	71·4	48·8	40·0	85·5	87·1
visits	M–H χ^2	13·9*		14·1*		1·5	
Age with	Education (years)						
survival	0	74·5	58·5	66·2	37·5	85·7	100·0
controlling	1–6	77·2	58·5	64·7	57·1	85·0	76·5
for	7+	73·5	33·3	60·3	80·0	81·9	85·9
education	M–H χ^2	14·1*		14·5*		0·7	
Age with	Residence						
survival	Urban	81·4	57·8	62·8	31·8	83·4	86·0
controlling	Rural	71·8	57·3	67·7	42·1	78·2	83·3
for	Slum	73·0	66·7	67·4	66·7	—	—
residence	M–H χ^2	11·7*		12·4*		0·9	
Age with	Smoking						
survival							
controlling	No	74·7	58·0	63·8	42·9	81·9	83·6
for	Yes	92·3	66·7	25·0	100·0	81·5	88·2
smoking	M–H χ^2	12·7*		11·4*		0·3	

† n in parentheses
‡ Mantel–Haenszel
* Significant at $\alpha = 0·05$, Pr (1 df χ^2⟨3·84⟩) = 0·05
% underlined are based on 5 cases or less

age is concerned. In two of the three hospitals, there is a strong relationship between maternal age and infant survival, but none between maternal age and low birth weight. In the other hospital, there is a moderate relationship between maternal age and low birth weight (although age is the least important of the explanatory variables examined), but none between maternal age and infant survival.

This work supports earlier conclusions that maternal age does influence the outcome of pregnancy. These conclusions are reinforced by showing that in the two developing countries, the relationship between age and infant survival and morbidity (as indicated by depressed Apgar scores) persists even when various social factors are controlled. Contrary to the findings of some other writers, no relationship was found between maternal age and birth weight, except in the Hungarian hospital where, although age explained some of the variance, other factors (especially smoking) predominated.

Perhaps the most important conclusion to be drawn from this analysis is that although maternal age does influence infant survival, in a population otherwise considered low risk and when the pregnancy is well-managed, the influence of age can be greatly reduced. Although Baird[1] found that maternal age differences remained (although less pronounced) in spite of increased intervention intended to eliminate them, the Hungarian data analyzed suggested that today (20 years after Baird's study) the technology exists to reduce the difference substantially among socioeconomically low-risk patients. The great majority of the patients delivering at the Hungarian hospital are relatively well-educated, receive good antenatal care and are of low parity; for these patients, age appears to be relatively unimportant. In the Mexican and Egyptian hospitals also, the difference between the older and younger women is at its smallest in the low-risk groups with maximum antenatal care, maximum education and medium parity.

Also emerging from this analysis is the fact that the older mothers contribute more than their share to perinatal mortality. In the Mexican hospital, for example (Table 7), mothers of 35 and older represent 22·6% of all the non-teenage mothers, yet 38·3% of the deaths occurring before discharge are to the infants of these mothers. In the Egyptian hospital, the contribution is even greater; older mothers constitute 16·6% of deliveries (to non-teenagers), but nearly twice that percentage (29·7%) of the identified perinatal deaths.

Since it is probable that a majority of the pregnancies to the women over 35 were unplanned, especially those at higher parities, it would

Table 7 Contribution of older mothers to the number of perinatal deaths compared with their contribution to the total number of births

	Mexico	Egypt	Hungary
Women 35+ years as % of all deliveries*	22·6	16·6	5·2
Deaths to infants of mothers 35+ as % of all early infant deaths*	38·3	29·7	6·5

* Teenaged mothers excluded, so percentages are higher than in Table 1

seem that older women would be particularly receptive to postpartum family planning. In the Mexican hospital, 80% of the older women state that they want no more children after this delivery; the comparable figures for Egypt and Hungary are 90% and 89%, respectively. Even among those older mothers whose babies died before discharge from the hospital, the percentages are 80, 85 and 68 for the three hospitals. Elimination of unplanned pregnancies after age 35 would not only significantly reduce the birth rate among these populations, but would have an even greater impact on perinatal mortality.

The impact of childbearing at advanced ages is great, both in terms of maternal and child health and in demographic terms. Table 1 shows the percentage of all births in Mexico, Egypt and Hungary to women 35 years old or more. In Mexico, more than one fifth and in Egypt almost one fourth of all births are to older women, compared with less than 5% in Hungary. Thus, simply by eliminating births to women over 35, Egypt could reduce its birth rate by 25%.

The contribution made by older mothers to maternal and perinatal mortality and morbidity is greater than the number of births would suggest, and elimination of childbearing beyond age 35 would significantly reduce mortality and morbidity.

References

1 Baird, D. (1963). The contribution of operative obstetrics to prevention of perinatal death. *J. Obstet. Gynaecol. Br. Commonw.* **70**, 204
2 Caspi, E. and Lifshitz, Y. (1979). Delivery at 40 years and over. *Is. J. Med. Sci.*, **15**, 418

3 Daniels, P. and Weingarten, K. (1979). A new look at the medical risks in late childbearing. *Women and Health*, **4**, 5

4 Grizzle, J. E., Starmer, F. C. and Koch, G. G. (1969). Analysis of categorical data by linear models. *Biometrics*, **25**, 489

5 Israel, S. L. and Deutschberger, J. (1964). Relation of the mother's age to obstetric performance. *Obstet. Gynecol. NY*, **24**, 411

6 Kajanoja, P. and Widholm, O. (1978). Pregnancy and delivery in women aged 40 and over. *Obstet. Gynecol. NY*, **51**, 47

7 Mantel, N. and Haenszel, W. (1959). Statistical aspects of the analysis of data from retrospective studies of disease. *J. Natl. Cancer Inst.*, **22**, 719

8 Morrison, I. (1975). The elderly primigravida. *Am. J. Obstet. Gynecol.*, **121**, 465

9 Namboodiri, N. K. and Balakrishnan, V. (1958–9). On the effect of maternal age and parity on the birth weight of the offspring (Indian infants). *Ann. Hum. Genet.*, **23**, 189

10 Nortman, D. (1974). Parental Age as a Factor in Pregnancy Outcome and Child Development. Reports on Population/Family Planning, No. 16. The Population Council, New York

11 Resseguie, L. J. (1977). The artifactual nature of effects on maternal age on risk of stillbirth. *J. Biosoc. Sci.*, **9**, 191

2
The development of an index of high-risk pregnancy

J. A. FORTNEY and E. W. WHITEHORNE

The concept of the high-risk pregnancy is important in obstetrics. The ability to predict the birth of a jeopardized infant before its delivery means that decisions about the optimal management of the pregnancy can be made, and the chances of a favorable outcome can be increased. Anderson and colleagues[3] have shown, for example, that neonatal morbidity is significantly reduced (and the cost of hospitalization approximately halved) if patients are referred *before* delivery rather than *after*.

Because this is so important, many attempts have been made to develop an index or score for classifying high-risk pregnancies. None of these, however, is entirely satisfactory, and much progress remains to be made in this area[17].

High-risk indices are most often developed on a rather arbitrary basis, variables are selected for inclusion on the basis of clinical judgment, and importance assigned to the variables in a similar fashion. Indices based on appropriate statistical analysis of a large number of births are free of the arbitrariness, but tend to be excessively complicated to administer, e.g. the index of Donahue and Wan[7].

At the present time, it appears that there remains a significant proportion of pregnancies for which a poor outcome unpredictably occurs. Rayburn and his colleagues[21] found that two thirds of distressed infants born at term were not predictable, and Lesinski[17] refers to the 'big unknown', i.e. the genetic factors of both parents and the fetus which makes prediction difficult if not impossible. Goodwin *et al.*[11] found that half of the deaths in the low-risk group were attributable to congenital malformations that are often difficult to predict.

A high-risk index is of no use if a significant proportion of high-risk patients are not diagnosed as such (false negative), or if a significant proportion of patients are defined as being at high risk when they are not (false positive).

In evaluating the usefulness of any diagnostic tool, the consequences of misdiagnosis must be considered. Often this depends on what kind of action is to be taken as a result of the diagnosis. Let us examine the consequences of error in classifying a patient.

The consequences of false negative results, (i.e. high-risk patients who are mistakenly classified as being at low risk), may be that a patient who needs special care does not receive it, which may result in increased mortality or morbidity for the mother and/or the baby. The consequences of a false positive assessment are that a patient who does not require additional care receives it, perhaps with the use of scarce resources that could be better used elsewhere; the patient may be referred to another hospital unnecessarily and may be subjected to unnecessary intervention. All of these consequences can be costly.

However, if the hospital is well-equipped, if anesthetists and pediatricians are routinely standing by, then the additional cost to both the patient and the hospital are minimal. If the patient would remain in the same hospital regardless of whether she is considered to be at high or low risk, then the inconvenience to the patient is minimal. If resources are abundant, use of them unnecessarily on a misclassified patient does not mean that they will not be available later for a correctly classified patient. However, in all of these situations, the possibility of unnecessary intervention remains.

Any diagnostic tool can be analytically evaluated in terms of five characteristics. These characteristics are defined mathematically in Table 1 and as follows:

(1) *False positive* refers to the situation in which patients are defined as having the condition, when in fact they do not (i.e. the obstetric patient who is classified as being at high risk, when she is not at risk).
(2) *False negative* refers to the situation in which patients with the condition are defined as being free from the condition (i.e. the high-risk obstetric patient is misclassified as being at low risk).
(3) *Sensitivity* refers to the ability of the test to find the condition in

Table 1   Definitions of the criteria of evaluation

| Actual | Diagnosis | | Total |
	At risk	Not at risk	
At risk	A	B	G
Not at risk	C	D	H
Total	E	F	

Sensitivity = A/G. Specificity = D/H
False positive = C/E. False negative = B/F
Rate = A/E

patients who are at high risk (i.e. the percentage of high-risk patients who are defined as being at high risk).

(4) *Specificity* refers to the ability of a test to define risk only where risk exists (i.e. the percentage of low-risk patients who are classified as being at low risk).

(5) *The rate* is that at which the predicted event occurs in patients classified as being at risk. (What percentage of obstetric patients classified as being at high risk actually have an adverse outcome of pregnancy?)

An improvement in any one of the factors necessarily occurs only at the expense of one or more of the others. For example, as the sensitivity increases, so does the rate of false positives; as the specificity increases (i.e. improves), so does the rate of false negatives. Thus, a factor in deciding the most appropriate cutpoint is an evaluation of the consequences of the different kinds of error. The physician or the hospital should decide in advance the negative consequences, in their own particular situation, of the false positives and of the false negatives.

Administrative preference might be to decrease the percentage of patients defined as being at risk (i.e. lower the sensitivity and false positives and increase the specificity and false negatives by raising the cutoff point), whereas a clinician might prefer to lower the cutoff point, thus increasing the sensitivity and false positives, and reducing the specificity and false negatives. Clearly, neither response is 'correct', and a trade-off must be made to arrive at the best judgment on balance.

As Table 2 shows, most risk assessment scores classify a rather high percentage of patients as being at risk. Sensitivity tends to be quite high and the number of false negatives tends to be low. Specificity, on the other hand, is rather low and the number of false positives is remarkably high – up to 96%. This is a conservative approach from the

Table 2 Performance of various risk assessment scores in predicting perinatal outcome

	Percent assessed at risk	Sensitivity	Specificity	False positive	False negative
Dependent variable = perinatal mortality					
Goodwin et al.[11]	14	77·8	97·1	17·0	4·0
Morrison et al.[18]	19	69·7	82·0	93·0	0·7
Akhtar et al.[2]					
(high and medium risk)	26	70·0	n.a.	n.a.	n.a.
Hobel et al.[14,15]	34	50·4	68·5	77·2	11·8
Edwards et al.[8]	47	88·6	54·5	93·7	0·7
Sokol et al.[22]*	49	84·2	52·1	94·9	0·9
Halliday et al.[13]					
(high and medium risk)	62	96·8	38·5	96·2	0·2
(high risk only)	16	67·7	75·0	93·6	1·1
Dependent variable = preterm birth					
Akhtar et al.[2](a)					
(high and medium risk)	26	43·6	76·7	79·4	9·2
(high risk only)	12	25·5	89·9	74·1	10·3
Creasey et al.[6](a)					
(high and medium risk)	32	79·7	70·9	84·9	1·8
(high risk only)	13	64·4	90·4	69·6	2·5
Nesbitt et al.[19](b)					
(high and medium risk)	69	78·1	31·5	92·6	4·6
(high risk only)	30	46·9	71·3	89·8	5·0
Dependent variable = low birthweight(c)					
Akhtar et al.[2]					
(high and medium risk)	26	38·7	76·2	80·0	11·0
(high risk only)	12	25·1	90·0	72·1	11·3
Nesbitt et al.[19]					
(high and medium risk)	69	76·5	32·6	85·2	10·0
(high risk only)	30	43·2	72·8	80·4	10·6
Dependent variable = depressed 5 minute Apgar Score					
Goodwin et al.[11](d)	14	67·3	97·9	19·5	4·1
Akhtar et al.[2](e)					
(high and medium risk)	26	55·2	76·5	84·8	4·3
(high risk only)	12	35·6	89·8	78·9	5·2

* Using Hobel's scoring system
(a) less than 37 weeks
(b) less than 36 weeks
(c) less than 2500 g
(d) less than 4
(e) less than 7

clinical point of view. Several of the high-risk scores shown in Table 2 are classified into three groups – high-, medium- and low-risk. The appropriate evaluation criteria are calculated with the medium group included among the high-risk patients and with the medium-risk patients included with the low-risk patients. The second situation, of course, corresponds to raising the cutoff point thereby improving specificity at the expense of sensitivity. Table 2 includes only those articles in the list of references from which the calculations could be made. A surprisingly large number of articles on this subject neither give the sensitivity, specificity or the percentage of misclassified cases, nor do they provide the reader with sufficient information to make those calculations.

The rather high rate of false positives brings us to a major problem inherent in the development of risk assessment scores. If the physician reacts appropriately to a high-risk assessment and manages the patient skillfully, then an unsatisfactory outcome of pregnancy is avoided, and the case is subsequently recorded as a misclassification (i.e. a false positive). Theoretically, this would be most true if the outcome variable of interest is perinatal mortality, less true if a depressed Apgar score is the outcome of interest, and least true if either low birth weight or low gestation are the outcomes of interest, since the physician is more easily able to influence survival than either weight or gestation.

In addition to its predictability, a high-risk score should be simple to administer. The index developed by Donahue and Wan[7] involved only nine variables, but each was given a 'factor value' to two decimal places and a 'weighting factor' to two decimal places which are then multiplied; the scores for the nine variables are added, and give a score with four decimal places. Hobel's score involves 51 prenatal factors and 40 intrapartum factors, each of which are scored 1–10[14,15]. It is not possible to calculate sensitivity or specificity from Donahue and Wan's[7] published data; in the case of Hobel and associates' data they are not particularly good (see Table 2). Thus, complexity does not necessarily contribute to accuracy of prediction. The method developed by Adelstein and Fedrick[1] uses ten risk factors, with scores on each factor ranging from $0\cdot4$ to $5\cdot9$ (not the same for each factor), and the individual scores are multiplied. Not enough information is given to calculate false negatives and positives, or specificity, but sensitivity appears to be a satisfactory 60% when 12% of the population is identified as being at high risk.

The most useful of the indices developed to date appears to be that of Goodwin and colleagues[11]. Twenty-seven factors are grouped into three categories; each of the three categories receives a score and the sum of the three ranges from 0 to 10. Although synergism is recognized by scoring 1 for a factor alone but 2 if the factor occurs simultaneously with another, the index does not permit recording more than two factors within a single category. The great value of Goodwin's index is that, with the test population used, only 14% of the population was defined as being at risk, which accounted for 77·8% of the perinatal deaths and 67·3% of the depressed Apgar scores (i.e. high sensitivity).

Much of the published work on the development of risk scores is conceptually confused (and confusing). The relevant outcome variables are often not clearly stated, and sometimes appear to be a combination of low birth weight, perinatal death, depressed Apgar score, and even maternal complications. Usually, the criteria by which the score will be judged are not clear; the most commonly used is the percentage of all perinatal deaths (or whatever the outcome variable is defined to be) that were defined as high risk.

Another source of confusion is the time at which the assessment is made. It is not useful to predict a poor outcome at a time when it is too late to change the treatment. A condition discovered intrapartum will not change the management of the pregnancy, although it may change the method of delivery. In some of the material published on this subject, the writers do not specify the time at which the assessment should be made, and even include some postpartum factors.

With these desirable characteristics in mind, we developed a model for a high-risk index, and tested this index on two large sets of data. The model was developed with the use of data collected from a random sample of hospitals in Colombia. The variables were selected for inclusion by a multiple discriminant analysis, and the weights were assigned to these variables by determining the relationship among the variables and scaling the proportions to integer weights. Finally, curves were plotted that showed the relationship among sensitivity and specificity, false positives and false negatives, and the rate of adverse outcome.

The adverse outcomes we selected for the model were (1) stillbirth or neonatal death before discharge from the hospital and (2) low birth weight (2500 g or less).

Nine factors in two categories were selected for inclusion in the score. The first five factors can be ascertained at any point during the pregnancy and require no tests and no clinical judgment to be made. These antepartum factors and their weights are as follows:

(1) *Mother's age.* Less than 16 years=2, 16–17 years=1, 18–29 years=0, 30–34 years=1, and 35+years=2.
(2) *Parity.* Nulliparity=1, parity 1–3=0, parity 4–6=1, and parity 7+=2. (Parity is defined as deliveries at 20 weeks or more, whether live or stillborn.)
(3) *Gravidity.* Nulligravidity=1, gravidity 1–3=0, gravidity 4–6=1, and gravidity 7+=2. (Gravidity is defined as live births, still-births, spontaneous and induced abortions.)
(4) *Poor obstetric history.* The number of previous stillbirths, spontaneous abortions and cesarean sections are added together; if the resulting sum is none, the score=0, if 1, the score=1, if more than 1 the score=2
(5) *Antepartum condition.* No pathologic condition during pregnancy is scored 0, *any* condition is scored 1

The other four factors are determined when the patient is admitted into the hospital for delivery, i.e. labor has already started. Again, all four factors require no tests being made; although clinical judgment is called for, the scores can easily be assigned by a midwife. The four intrapartum factors are as follows:

(6) *Number of antenatal visits made.* None or 1 visit=2, 2–5 visits=1, 6+ visits=0
(7) *Presentation.* If the presentation is vertex, occiput anterior the score=0, any other presentation is scored 1
(8) *Duration of labor.* No labor (i.e. elective cesarean section or precipitate delivery) is scored 1, up to 18 hours is scored 0, more than 18 hours is scored 1
(9) *Estimated gestation.* 20–27 weeks=5, 28–35 weeks=4, 36–39 weeks=1, 40–42 weeks=0, 43 weeks or more=1

Adding the scores of the individual factors produces an index that ranges from 0 to 9 when the antepartum factors alone are added, and from 0 to 18 when the combined antepartum and intrapartum factors are added. Multiplying the scores (which would give added weight to factors held in combination by permitting interaction between two or more factors) did not produce a better index in terms of predictive value. The combined antepartum and intrapartum factors produced a better index in terms of predictive value than did the antepartum factors alone.

Figure 1A–F shows the five criteria by which the index is evaluated, for the antepartum index alone, and for the antepartum and intra-partum parts combined. Since other writers[7] have found that it is more difficult to identify high risk among nulliparous women than among parous women, Figure 1 also shows the two indices for nulliparous

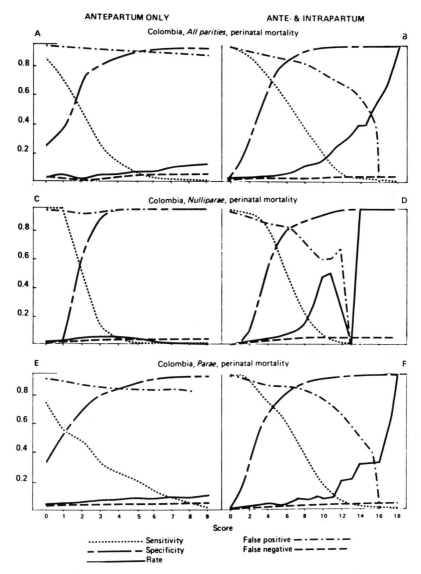

ANTEPARTUM ONLY   ANTE- & INTRAPARTUM

A   Colombia, *All parities*, perinatal mortality   B

C   Colombia, *Nulliparae*, perinatal mortality   D

E   Colombia, *Parae*, perinatal mortality   F

Score

.... Sensitivity   False positive — · — · — · —
— ·· — · Specificity   False negative — — — — —
————Rate

Figure 1 Five statistical criteria used to evaluate an antepartum and an ante- and intrapartum index of high risk of perinatal mortality before hospital discharge. Data from Colombia

women (C and D) and for multiparous women (E and F) separately. In Figure 1, the outcome of interest is perinatal death before hospital discharge; the data are from Colombia. (Tables showing the data used to generate the graphs may be obtained by writing to the authors.)

Figure 1A shows the antepartum part of the index. This part of the index alone does not predict well; the death rate at the higher scores is close to zero, and is highest in the middle scores. False positives remain high at all levels of the score, and the sensitivity is quite poor. Adding in the intrapartum part of the index produces much better results (B); the correspondence between increasing death rate and increasing score on the index is good and achieves 100% at the highest score. The false positives decline, particularly after a score of 8. Since the death rate before discharge is a low 2·8%, it is inevitable that false negatives remain low at all levels of the score. Sensitivity and specificity are optimal at a score of 5.

Suppose, after examining Figure 1B, we decided that a score of 5 is an appropriate cutoff at which to define patients as being at high risk, i.e. if a woman has a score of 6 or higher she will receive some kind of special attention. This would mean that 38·1% of all women would be classified as being at high risk, and that 68·9% of all the deaths before discharge would have been predicted (sensitivity). However, 91·6% of those classified as being at high risk would not have had an adverse outcome of pregnancy (false positives). On the other hand, 77·6% of the low-risk patients would have been correctly identified (specificity). By raising the cutoff just one point to 6 (i.e. 7 or higher is high risk) and by classifying less than a fourth (23·8%) of the women as being at high risk, we can still account for more than half (56·1%) of all deaths (sensitivity). False positives are lowered to 88·8% (which is still high), and false negatives increase only to 1·5%; 86·7% of the low-risk women are correctly identified (specificity).

Comparing the results for the parous and the nulliparous women for the combined antepartum and intrapartum index (Figures 1D and F, we find that there is remarkably little difference in the predictive value of the index for the two groups of women. The curves in Figures 1D and F are quite similar except that they become erratic at the higher scores for nulliparous women, primarily because the numbers are small. Taking the same cutoff point of 5, we find that the sensitivity is 66·9% for nulliparous women and 69·9% for parous women; specificity is 78·6% for nulliparous women and 76·9% for parous women; false positives are 92·6% and 91·0%, respectively, and false negatives are

1·1% and 1·3%, respectively. Even the percentages of women classified as being at high risk in the two groups – 22·5% of nulliparous women and 24·6% of parous women – are very similar.

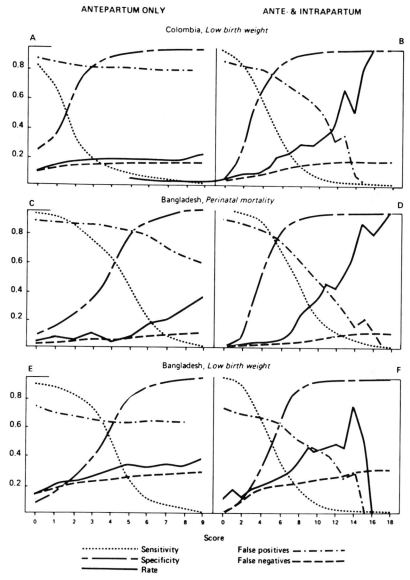

ANTEPARTUM ONLY   **ANTE- & INTRAPARTUM**

Colombia, *Low birth weight*

Bangladesh, *Perinatal mortality*

Bangladesh, *Low birth weight*

Score

·········· Sensitivity	False positives — · — · — · —
– — Specificity	False negatives — — — — —
—— Rate	

Figure 2 Five statistical criteria used to evaluate antepartum and an ante- and intra-partum index of high risk of perinatal mortality before hospital discharge and high risk of low birth weight. Data from Colombia and Bangladesh

Figure 2 shows the antepartum-only index and the combined ante-partum and intrapartum index for all women in which the outcome of interest is birth weight (i.e. the probability of weight being 2500 g or less). Figure 2A and B show data for Colombia, whereas the other four panels show the equivalents of Figure 1A and B and Figure 2A and B for Bangladesh.

In a general way, perhaps the most apparent fact in Figure 1 is that in the three graphs on the right (i.e. those for the combined antepartum and intrapartum scores) the line that represents the proportion with the outcome of interest shows a much more pronounced upward trend than is the case with the antepartum index alone. This confirms our conclusion from Figure 1 that the combined score is a much better predictor than the antepartum score alone. The next important fact to notice is that only with the combined index does the curve representing false positives decline very substantially. This confirms the statement by Rayburn and colleagues[21] that it is difficult to predict which infants are threatened until labor has begun.

The similarities between the results for the two countries are quite surprising, given how different the two settings are. If we take perinatal death before maternal discharge as an example, in Colombia 2·9% of babies died before maternal discharge; in Bangladesh, the per-centage was 8·1%. Sensitivity and specificity were optimized at a score of 5 in Colombia and 6 in Bangladesh; at that score, sensitivity and specificity averaged 73·2% in Colombia and 76·5% in Bangladesh; and at that point 23·8% of the Colombian women and 23·3% of the Bangladeshi women were classified as being at high risk. If we look at low birth weight instead of perinatal death, 12·1% of the Colombian babies weighed 2500 g or less compared with 23·6% of the Bangladeshi babies; sensitivity and specificity were optimized at 4 in Colombia and at 5 in Bangladesh (both one point lower than the optimal score for perinatal death), and at that point sensitivity and specificity averaged 62·1% in Colombia and 60·0% in Bangladesh, and 38·1% of the women were classified as being at high risk in Colombia and 37·0% in Bangladesh.

The five statistical criteria are affected by the incidence of the outcome variable in the population. In Bangladesh, for example, 8·1% of the infants died before maternal discharge, and 23·6% of the infants weighed 2500 g or less. Sensitivity is much higher at all scores for death than it is for low birth weight; specificity, on the other hand, is almost identical at each score. False positives are higher with the rarer outcome (death), and false negatives are lower at each level of the score. The incidence at each score is obviously higher, the higher the overall incidence.

Although many high-risk indices have been developed, a great deal of work remains to be done. Also, it may be true that we are asking too much of the high-risk index; there are too many conflicting demands. It is impossible to keep both false positives and false negatives low, as specificity increases, sensitivity inevitably decreases. It is impossible to keep small the percentage classified as being at high risk and at the same time predict a large percentage of the jeopardized babies.

Nevertheless, it is possible to make a sensible classification of obstetric patients based on the score of a high-risk index as long as consideration has been given to expected rates of error and the consequences of error. It must be accepted that error is inevitable; therefore, decisions need to be made as to the most acceptable type of error that allows for maximum use of available resources. Risk indices can contribute greatly to the overall management of high-risk pregnancy by providing a mechanism for coarse screening. Finer screening by clinical testing can then be used to maximize the allocation of often scarce resources and positively influence the outcome of the pregnancy.

References

1 Adelstein, P., Fedrick, J. (1978). Antenatal identification of women at increased risk of being delivered of a low birth weight infant at term. *Br. J. Obstet. Gynaecol.*, **85**, 8

2 Akhtar, J., Sehgal, N. N. (1980). Prognostic value of a prepartum and intrapartum risk-scoring method. *South. Med. J.*, **73**, 411

3 Anderson, C. L., Aladjem, S., Ayuste, O., Caldwell, C., Ismail, M. (1981). An analysis of maternal transport within a suburban metropolitan region. *Am. J. Obstet. Gynecol.*, **140**, 499

4 Aubry, R. H., Pennington, J. C. (1973). Identification and evaluation of high-risk pregnancy: the perinatal concept. *Clin. Obstet. Gynecol.*, **16**, 3

5 Coopland, A. T., Peddle, L. J., Baskett, T. F. *et al.* (1977). A simplified antepartum high-risk pregnancy scoring form. *Can. Med. Assoc. J.*, **116**, 999

6 Creasey, R. K., Gummer, B. A., Liggins, G. C. (1980). System for predicting spontaneous preterm birth. *Obstet. Gynecol.*, **55**, 692

7 Donahue, C. L., Wan, T. T. H. (1973). Measuring obstetric risks of prematurity: a preliminary analysis of neonatal death. *Am. J. Obstet. Gynecol.*, **116**, 911

8 Edwards, L. E., Barrada, I., Tatreau, R. W., Hakanson, E. Y. (1979). A simplified antepartum risk scoring system. *Obstet. Gynecol.*, **54**, 237

9 Foy, J. E., Backes, C. R. (1978). A study of the relationship between Goodwin's

high-risk scoring system and fetal outcome. *J. Am. Med. Assoc.*, **78**, 113

10 Fedrick, J. (1976). Antenatal identification of women at risk of spontaneous pre-term birth. *Br. J. Obstet. Gynaecol.*, **83**, 351

11 Goodwin, J. W., Dunne, J. T., Thomas, B. W. (1969). Antepartum identification of the fetus at risk. *Can. Med. Assoc. J.*, **101**, 57

12 Haeri, A. D., South, J., Naldrett, J. (1974). A scoring system for identifying patients with a high risk of perinatal mortality. *J. Obstet. Gynaecol. Br. Commonw.*, **81**, 535

13 Halliday, H. L., Jones, P. K., Jones, S. L. (1980). Method of screening obstetric patients to prevent reproductive wastage. *Obstet. Gynecol.*, **55**, 656

14 Hobel, C. J., Hyvarinen, M. A., Okada, D. M., Oh, W. (1973). Prenatal and intrapartum high-risk screening. *Am. J. Obstet. Gynecol.*, **117**, 1

15 Hobel, C. J. (1978). Risk Assessment in Perinatal Medicine. In Makowski, E. L. (ed.) *Clinical Obstetrics and Gynecology*, p. 287. (New York: Harper and Row, Inc)

16 Jones, P. K., Halliday, J. L., Jones, S. L. (1979). Prediction of neonatal deaths or need for interhospital transfer by prenatal risk characteristics of mother. *Med. Care*, **17**, 796

17 Lesinski, J. (1975). High risk pregnancy: unresolved problems of screening, management and prognosis. *Obstet. Gynecol.*, **45**, 599

18 Morrison, I., Olsen, J. (1979). Perinatal mortality and antepartum risk scoring. *Obstet. Gynecol.*, **53**, 362

19 Nesbitt, R. E. L. Jr., Aubry, R. H. (1969). High risk obstetrics. II. Value of semi-objective grading system in identifying the vulnerable groups. *Am. J. Obstet. Gynecol.*, **103**, 972

20 Pavelka, R., Riss, P., Parschalk, O., Reinold, E. (1980). Practical experiences in the prevention of prematurity using Thalhammer's score. *J. Perinat. Med.*, **8**, 100

21 Rayburn, W. F., Anderson, C. W., O'Shaughnessy, R. W., Rickman, W. P. (1981). Predictability of the distressed term infant. *Am. J. Obstet. Gynecol.*, **140**, 489

22 Sokol, R. J., Rosen, M. G., Stojkov, J., Chik, L. (1977). Clinical application of high risk scoring on an obstetric service. *Am. J. Obstet. Gynecol.*, **128**, 652

23 Sogbanmu, M. O. (1979). Perinatal mortality and maternal mortality in General Hospital, Ondo, Nigeria. Use of high-risk pregnancy predictive scoring index. *Niger. Med. J.*, **9**, 123

3
Improving obstetric care by training traditional birth attendants, Fortaleza, Brazil

G. ARAUJO, L. ARAUJO, B. JANOWITZ, S. L. WALLACE and
M. POTTS

More than half the babies delivered into the world are not attended by a trained midwife or doctor. Several projects have attempted to upgrade the performance of the traditional birth attendants (TBAs) who assist a large number of these deliveries. Such schemes usually involve three inputs: basic training in delivery procedures, provision of some type of equipment, and a system of referring women thought to be at high risk for obstetric complications to institutional settings. A pilot scheme in the rural areas surrounding the city of Fortaleza in northeastern Brazil was implemented in 1975. This program was developed to improve maternal and infant health care using previously untrained local personnel and limited resources. The program is unusual in that not only do TBAs receive basic training in obstetrics, but they also deliver women in small maternity centers provided by their communities instead of in the woman's home.

The northeast of Brazil is the poorest region of the country, with a *per capita* income of less than half that of the country as a whole. The region's infant mortality rate (142) is higher than that for any other region and typical of countries at low levels of development. Ceara, a state in this region, has a population of approximately 5·3 million, of which 25% live in its capital city, Fortaleza. Health resources are extremely limited, with a population-to-physician ratio of approximately 3000 : 1 compared with 1500 : 1 for Brazil as a whole. While an estimate of the proportion of deliveries attended in hospitals in Ceara is not available, data from neighboring states show that about 75% of deliveries occur in hospitals. The proportion of hospital deliveries is lower in rural areas (59%) than in major urban areas such as Fortaleza (96%) or in smaller urban areas (85%).

THE TRADITIONAL BIRTH ATTENDANT

The TBA of northeastern Brazil is typically a middle-aged woman who in the past has been asked to help neighbors or friends at the time of delivery. After numerous such experiences she becomes recognized as a midwife in her community. She acquires her knowledge from her own experiences and observations or from information handed down from her mother or received from her colleagues. Most TBAs are illiterate but have a keen sense of the practical and the obvious. At delivery, the TBA almost always maintains her patient in a sitting or squatting position during the expulsion period (usually 10–15 minutes), using low benches or birthing stools. The baby is put to the breast immediately after delivery, even before the cord is cut.

THE URBAN, UNIVERSITY-BASED HOSPITAL

The Assis Chateaubriand Teaching Maternity Hospital (MEAC), one of only two free maternity hospitals in Fortaleza, is part of the medical school of the Federal University of Ceara. This 150-bed hospital, the largest in the city, has about 8000 deliveries a year and provides the most sophisticated obstetric care in the area. Approximately 30 000 women are seen each year through its outpatient department in antenatal, postpartum, family planning, and gynecological cancer prevention clinics. Hospital staff have been concerned for many years with the need to develop a rural health care delivery system to help poor women in surrounding rural areas who lack formal medical attention.

INTEGRATION OF TBAs AND THE HOSPITAL

The impetus for developing a system for meeting the maternity care needs of the rural poor came from the senior author's observation that each year seven or eight women from the area surrounding the village of Guaiuba were dying in childbirth at MEAC. It was felt that if maternity care could be improved in the area, maternal mortality would decrease. After several discussions with community leaders, support was enlisted in recruiting local TBAs to participate in a program to upgrade their skills. In addition, the community leaders offered the use of a vacant building to serve as an obstetric unit.

A 3-month practical and theoretical course was given at MEAC for the TBAs. After the course, the best of them were put to work in the unit. The others were sent back to the community to continue their work at the home level with general instructions for referral of high-risk pregnancies.

After the success of the project in Guaiuba, other communities in the area requested assistance in setting up similar projects. To date, there are approximately 15 free-standing obstetric units.

These obstetric units each have an outpatient clinic, a delivery room, and a room with two to seven beds for postpartum recovery. They are furnished with rather simple equipment: obstetric and clinical stethoscopes, sphygmomanometers, adult and infant weighing scales, and occasionally, reactive strips and saline solution for intravenous infusions. The obstetric units are open to the community every day of the week, 24 hours a day with at least one trained TBA always on duty. An ambulance and driver, provided by the rural social security insurance program, are available at all times to transport women with delivery complications to MEAC.

A team of one obstetrician and one nurse from MEAC visit each of the units twice a week to supervise the TBA's activities and provide antenatal care for high-risk patients. Patients to be included in the high-risk group are selected by applying an antenatal risk index based on scoring of age, parity, previous pregnancy outcome, birth interval and socio-economic status. Patients are classified as being at high, medium or low risk.

Funding for the project is primarily provided by the Brazilian social security system, which pays the salaries of all employees of the obstetric units. Salaries of the visiting physician and nurse are paid by MEAC. Operating costs for the obstetric units range from US$200 per

month for the small units to US$2000 per month for the larger units.
The basic questions addressed by the present study are:

(1) How do deliveries by TBAs at the obstetric units compare with
    hospital deliveries in terms of maternal and infant morbidity and
    mortality?
(2) Do TBAs recognize high-risk patients and make appropriate
    referrals?
(3) What are the factors affecting the decision to refer a patient? Do
    TBAs refer the appropriate patients or should they refer more or
    fewer or different types of patients?
(4) Do complication rates suggest additional areas of training for
    TBAs or services that can be provided to improve perinatal and
    maternal health?

Data were obtained on women delivering at four obstetric units, one
located in a semi-urban area just outside Fortaleza (Lagoa Redonda)
and the other three in rural areas (Aguiraz, Guaiuba and Antonio
Diogo), and on women transferred to MEAC from these obstetric
units. The study was carried out over the 10-month period from
October 1980 to July 1981. Records were obtained for 1646 women
delivering at the obstetric units and for 235 women referred for
delivery from the units to MEAC.

The Maternity Record Summary form was used to collect
information for women delivering at the obstetric units and for
patients referred to MEAC. Women who were transferred to MEAC
received a transfer slip from the referring obstetric unit indicating the
reason(s) for their referral. A Maternity Record was completed for the
transferred women at MEAC. Data collection activities were
supervised at the obstetric units by two nurses who were responsible
for aiding the TBAs in the completion of the forms. At MEAC, data
collection was supervised by a physician.

The original study design was to include domiciliary deliveries by
TBAs (both trained and untrained) using a pictorial record. The
inclusion of deliveries by these TBAs would have allowed a more
comprehensive evaluation of the impact of training. However, since
the number of forms received was well below the estimated number of
births in the area, we were reasonably certain that we did not have
records for all deliveries. Without knowing whether the deliveries for
which we did have records were a 'random sample' of all TBA
deliveries, these data were not interpretable. Our experience in

attempting to collect records on home deliveries should caution other investigators concerning the difficulties of such a project.

FACTORS REFLECTING REFERRAL

Table 1 shows the number of women presenting at each of the four obstetric units and the percentage of women referred to MEAC for delivery from each of these units. The greatest number of women presented at Lagoa Redonda and the smallest at Antonio Diogo. The percentage of women referred to MEAC was highest at Guaiuba and lowest at Antonio Diogo, the unit furthest from Fortaleza.

The referral of women to MEAC was thought to be associated with factors such as age, parity, education, and antenatal problems (Table 2). Almost 30% of women over 40 years of age and 20% of those

Table 1 Percent referred by location of obstetric unit

	Total cases	Percent referred before delivery*	Travel time to MEAC (in minutes)
Lagoa Redonda	777	11·1	20
Aguiraz	578	13·5	30
Guaiuba	411	16·8	60
Antonio Diogo	115	1·7	90
Total	1881	12·5	

* Ten women who delivered at the obstetric units were later transferred to MEAC for treatment of postpartum problems

women with six or more previous live births were referred. However, there was very little difference in referral rates between women with no schooling and those who had some education.

As anticipated, women with antenatal problems were far more likely to have been referred than women who had no problems. Over 95% of women with antepartum hemorrhage or hypertensive disorders were referred, and all women with reported premature rupture of the membranes were referred.

The data show that almost 25% of the women presenting at the obstetric units were designated as being at high risk (risk index ≥5). Twenty percent of these women were referred to MEAC for delivery.

Table 2   Characteristics and antenatal status of women presenting at obstetric units and percent referred

	Total		% Referred for delivery
Age (years)			
<20	20·9	(392)	12·0
20–29	52·4	(986)	9·3
30–39	22·1	(415)	16·9
40+	4·6	(87)	28·7
Total	100·0	(1880)	
Parity			
0	29·2	(549)	12·9
1–3	37·7	(710)	9·2
4–5	14·1	(265)	10·6
6+	19·0	(357)	19·9
Total	100·0	(1881)	
Education			
None	35·4	(665)	14·6
1–4 years	56·1	(1054)	11·3
5+ years	8·6	(161)	11·2
Total	100·0	(1880)	
Antenatal problems			
None	93·9	(1766)	7·0
Hemorrhage	1·1	(20)	95·0
Hypertensive disorders	3·8	(71)	95·8
Premature rupture of membranes	0·8	(15)	100·0
Other	0·5	(9)	100·0
Total	100·0	(1881)	
Risk index			
High (5+)	23·6	(444)	19·6
Medium (3–4)	13·9	(262)	15·3
Low (<3)	62·4	(1173)	9·2
Total	100·0	(1879)	

Nearly two thirds (62%) of the women were designated as being at low risk (risk index <3) and only 9% of them were referred to MEAC for delivery. As the purpose of the risk index was to determine which women were to be scheduled for prenatal care with a doctor or nurse

Table 3 Labor characteristics of women presenting at obstetric units and percent referred

	Total cases		% Referred for delivery
Presentation during labor			
Vertex, occiput anterior			
posterior or transverse	95·6	(1816)	10·9
Brow/face	1·1	(21)	28·6
Breech	1·8	(34)	61·8
Transverse	0·5	(9)	100·0
Compound	0·0	((1)	100·0
Total	100·0	(1881)	
Complications of labor/delivery			
None	96·5	(1815)	9·7
Prolonged/obstructed labor	2.3	(44)	97·7
Placenta previa	0·4	(7)	100·0
Placenta abruptio	0·4	(7)	85·7
Other	0·4	(8)	37·5
Total	100·0	(1881)	
Condition of fetus/neonate			
Normal	96·3	(1811)	9·9
Fetal distress	3·1	(59)	83·1
Other	0·5	(10)	60·0
Total	100·0	(1880)	

and not for determining referral, it is interesting to note that the probability of referral is still positively related to the risk index score.

Referral rates were much higher among women with abnormal presentations during labor than among women with cephalic presentations (Table 3). Women who had problems of labor and/or delivery, including prolonged or obstructed labor, placenta previa or placenta abruptio were much more frequently referred than women who had no problems. In addition, 83% of the reported cases of fetal distress during labor were referred as compared with only 10% of the cases when the condition of the fetus was normal.

DELIVERY (Table 4, columns 1–3)

All of the women delivering at the obstetric units had spontaneous deliveries, while 22% of the women referred to MEAC required

Table 4 Type of delivery and attendant by place of delivery and referral status for women presenting at obstetric units and at MEAC

	Presenting at obstetric units					
	Delivered at obstetric units	Referred to MEAC	All cases		Presenting at MEAC*	
Type of delivery						
Spontaneous (including breech extraction)	100·0	78·3	97·3	(1830)	89·7	(4492)
Forceps (low, mid, high)	0·0	3·8	0·5	(9)	1·6	(79)
Cesarean section	0·0	17·9	2·2	(42)	8·6	(432)
Total	100·0	100·0	100·0	(1881)	100·0	(5003)
Attendant at delivery						
Traditional birth attendant	99·6	0·0	87·2	(1639)	0·0	(0)
Student nurse	0·0	18·3	2·3	(43)	27·5	(1374)
Nurse	0·1	1·7	0·3	(5)	1·5	(76)
Medical student	0·0	16·2	2·0	(38)	21·1	(1057)
Physician	0·1	63·8	8·0	(151)	49·8	(2492)
None	0·2	0·0	0·2	(4)	0·1	(6)
Total	100·0	100·0	100·0	(1880)	100·0	(5005)

* Excludes private patients and referrals

operative intervention (4% were assisted with forceps – low/mid/high – and 18% were delivered by cesarean section).

All but six of the women delivered at the obstetric units were attended by TBAs. Four had no attendant and the other two were delivered by a nurse and a physician. Nearly two thirds (64%) of the women referred to MEAC were delivered by physicians, 16% were delivered by medical students and 20% had nurses or student nurses in attendance.

OUTCOME OF DELIVERY (Table 5, columns 1–3)

Almost 98% of the women delivered babies who were alive at discharge. The stillbirth rate was 18 per 1000 deliveries and five babies per 1000 born alive died before discharge. As anticipated, both the still-

Table 5 Outcome of delivery by place of delivery and referral status for women presenting at obstetric units and at MEAC

	Presenting at obstetric units				Presenting at MEAC*	
	Delivered at obstetric units	Referred to MEAC	Total			
Neonatal status						
Alive at discharge	99·2	87·2	97·7	(1838)	94·1	(4711)
Stillbirth	0·7	9·4	1·8	(33)	3·6	(182)
Postpartum death	0·1	3·4	0·5	(10)	2·3	(113)
Total	100·0	100·0	100·0	(1881)	100·0	(5006)
Birth weight						
< 2500 g	4·1	14·2	5·3	(99)	9·4	(465)
2500 + g	95·9	85·8	94·7	(1782)	90·6	(4465)
Total	100·0	100·0	100·0	(1881)	100·0	(4930)
5-minute Apgar score						
< 7	1·4	14·9	2·9	(53)	5·3	(253)
7–10	98·6	85·1	97·1	(1793)	94·7	(4480)
Total	100·0	100·0	100·0	(1846)	100·0	(4733)
Puerperal condition						
Normal	99·7	95·7	99·2	(1866)	98·0	(4908)
Fever	0·1	2·1	0·3	(6)	0·7	(34)
Bleeding	0·2	0·4	0·3	(5)	0·7	(37)
Other	0·0	1·7	0·2	(4)	0·5	(27)
Total	100·0	100·0	100·0	(1881)	100·0	(5006)

* Excludes private patients and referrals

birth rate and the rate of death before discharge were much higher for referred patients than for those delivered at the units. Almost 13% of the infants born to women referred to MEAC were not discharged alive, while less than 1% of those born to women delivering at the units died before discharge.

The percentage of low-birth-weight babies (< 2500 g) was much higher among the transferred women, as was the percentage of babies with a 5-minute Apgar score under 7. The percentage of women with some puerperal problem was low in both groups, but it was higher among the referred women. There were no maternal deaths among women delivering at the obstetric units or at MEAC.

The TBA training project achieved its primary goal of safer delivery for rural women. This evaluation demonstrates that TBAs with little or no formal education can be trained to refer high-risk women for hospital delivery while conducting safe deliveries in their own communities. To evaluate the performance of TBAs, we compared the birth outcome of women presenting to the TBAs with those of women presenting at MEAC (excluding private patients and all referrals).

The age distribution of women in the MEAC group is similar to that of the women presenting at the obstetric units (TBA group), with comparable percentages of women in the youngest (<20 years) and the oldest (40+ years) age categories. The women in the two groups were also of similar parity. However, women presenting at MEAC were more likely to have had some schooling (83%) than those in the TBA group (65%).

The two groups were comparable in terms of presentation of the fetus during labor, with 5% of the women in the TBA group having an abnormal presentation, as compared with 6% in the MEAC group. In the TBA group, however, only 4% of the women were reported as having complications of labor and/or delivery, compared to 9% in the MEAC group. Similarly, a higher percentage of women in the MEAC group were reported to have antenatal problems (18%) than in the TBA group (5%). These latter two findings may be partially explained by the tendency of traditional birth attendants to not record problems they consider to be usual or not serious.

These findings indicate that when comparisons are limited to variables that do not require interpretation by the attendant (e.g. age, parity, education, presentation), the two groups were comparable with, if anything, the MEAC group having a slight advantage.

No maternal deaths were seen in this review of 1881 women either delivered in obstetric units or referred to MEAC for delivery. In a similar group of women delivering at MEAC, three of 5006 patients died. This group includes nonprivate patients who had not been referred from other hospitals.

The stillbirth rate in the group of women who presented at the obstetric units (including women delivered at those units and those referred to MEAC) was 18 per 1000 deliveries, half the rate for the comparable MEAC group (Table 5, columns 3 and 4). In addition, the percentage of babies who died before leaving the hospital was much lower for women presenting at the TBA group than for the comparable MEAC group (0·5 compared to 2·3). These indices reflect, however, not only the ability of the TBAs to deal with normal deliveries and the effectiveness of the referral system but also differences in the health status of two populations. One indicator of the difference in health status between women in the two groups is the percentage of low-birth-weight babies. This percentage was lower for the TBA group (5·3%) than the MEAC group (9·4%).

In nearly all cases, TBAs were able to identify and refer women determined to be at above-average risk for delivery. A small group of women were referred and later diagnosed at MEAC as having no problem (for example, six women were referred for malpresentations but were reported to have cephalic presentations at delivery). Over-referral is probably preferable to a situation in which women with problems are not referred, although unnecessary referrals place an added strain on already scarce hospital resources, and monopolize the ambulance that might be needed for more urgent cases.

It might be expected that obstetric units further from MEAC would be less likely to refer patients because of the longer travel time necessary to reach the hospital. While Antonio Diogo, the obstetric unit furthest from MEAC, did have the lowest referral rate, the reason for this was more likely the availability of other, closer hospitals than its distance from MEAC. A more detailed analysis of patterns of referral is planned.

In an area such as northeast Brazil where health resources are very scarce, training women who already are active in delivering obstetric care is an efficient way of upgrading the obstetric care received by women in rural areas and an important step in the improvement of health services in seriously disadvantaged locations. Such a system can greatly extend the coverage provided by a hospital for very little extra cost. For example, whereas only 10% of women presenting at the obstetric units were delivered by physicians or medical students, 71% in the group presenting at MEAC were delivered by such highly trained personnel. In addition, only 2·2% of the women presenting at the obstetric units were delivered by cesarean as compared with 8·6% in the MEAC group.

Overall, the use of TBAs in this region points the way to an achievable, cost-effective improvement of obstetric services in a developing country with limited health budgets and severe shortages of trained midwives and physicians. It also points to the need for simple continuous evaluation of rural health services so that such problems can be identified and dealt with using whatever resources are available. Significantly, the communities themselves contributed resources to the improvement of health care by making available the buildings in which the TBAs work. The co-operation of the community is an important ingredient in the success of the program.

The success of this program has led to its expansion to include facilities for delivery at the homes of the trained TBAs. Currently there are plans for 25 one-bed units attached to the homes of the TBAs where women from the most remote communities can deliver their babies. This innovation brings good maternity care to a larger number of rural women who found delivery at a distant maternity hospital impractical, and should serve as an example of how health care in other parts of the world can be improved with community participation and low cost.

Section II:
CESAREAN DELIVERY

4

Cesarean delivery in selected Latin American hospitals

B. JANOWITZ, D. COVINGTON, J. E. HIGGINS, L. F. MORENO,
M. S. NAKAMURA, J. A. NUNEZ and M. M. LETELIER

Recent years have witnessed an increased incidence of cesarean delivery in many European countries and in the United States, where estimates of 15·2% in 1978 are up from 5·5% in 1970[3]. Much less is known about these rates elsewhere, particularly in the developing world.

This chapter examines selected factors that affect variations in cesarean birth rates in Central and South America. The impact of socio–demographic and medical indicators is considered, as is the mix of emergency and elective cesareans by hospital. Finally, the resource costs of cesarean and vaginal delivery are compared.

Table 1 shows the wide variation in rates of cesarean birth for participating hospitals reporting at least 1000 deliveries. The lowest of these is for a hospital in San Pedro Sula, Honduras (2·8%), and the highest for one in Campinas, Brazil (49·1%). This disparity in rates is probably the reflection of cultural conditions specific to a particular country, including patient and physician preferences and the hospital type studied, including financial arrangements for care.

Data for four of the hospitals cited in Table 1 are analyzed in detail. The basic criteria for selection were size of data base (large enough to permit detailed analyses) and rate of cesarean delivery (a wide range was desired). The hospitals are in Tegucigalpa, Honduras (rate, 4·9%, similar to the USA's in 1970), Cumaná, Venezuela (rate, 11·8%, similar to the USA's in 1976), Santiago, Chile (rate, 21·6%, currently above the USA's) and Campinas, Brazil (rate, 41·3%, markedly above the USA's)[2]. The stillbirth and maternal mortality rates reported by these hospitals are shown in Table 2.

The Brazilian maternity hospital is a large facility, whose paying patients defray the cost of their care out of pocket or private insurance. The majority of patients have their costs covered through the social security system, and the remainder are indigent with no medical coverage. The large general teaching hospital in Chile is reimbursed mainly through its public insurance coverage, though there are private

Table 1 Percentage cesarean delivery in selected hospitals in Latin America

County and city	Dates of study	Number of cases	Percentage cesarean delivery
Central America			
Costa Rica	7/77–2/78	2399	20·0
El Salvador			
San Salvador 1	3/77–6/77	1470	7·1
San Salvador 2	1/77–6/78	10358	6·0
Honduras			
San Pedro Sula	1/77–10/79	10358	2·8
Tegucigalpa	11/77–9/79	8258	4·9
Mexico	4/77–1/80	7089	13·2
Panama	7/77–6/78	9891	9·5
South America			
Brazil			
Campinas 1	9/77–4/79	6416	41·3
Campinas 2	9/77–3/79	2701	49·1
Chile			
Arica	4/77–6/79	6682	17·9
Santiago 1	12/77–6/78	5939	21·6
Santiago 2	5/77–1/78	3998	20·1
Valdivia	4/77–6/79	4973	19·5
Colombia*			
Type of hospital			
University	3/77–12/78	4122	8·5
University maternity	—	1402	6·8
Social Security	—	1501	6·5
Large general	—	1965	5·8
Medium general	—	2238	9·4
Small general	—	2802	9·2
Venezuela			
Cumaná	8/78–6/80	13586	11·8

* Random sample of hospitals

Table 2 Selected indices of mortality and time in hospital for four hospitals in Latin America

	Tegucigalpa, Honduras			Cuminá, Venezuela			Santiago, Chile			Campinas, Brazil		
	Total	Vaginal	Cesarean	Total	Vaginal	Cesarean	Total	Vaginal	Cesarean	Total	Vaginal	Cesarean
Number of cases	8258	7850	408 (4·9%)	13 586	11 987	1599 (11·8%)	5939	4656	1283 (21·6%)	6416	3763	2653 (41·3%)
Stillbirth rate per 1000 births	12·94	12·87	14·39	18·06	14·72	42·81	13·34	14·28	9·97	9·55	12·37	5·56
Maternal mortality per 1000	0·12	0·13	0	0·59	0·33	2·50	0·34	0·21	0·78	0	0	0
Medium nights hospitalized postpartum	1·0	1·0	6·0	1·0	1·0	4·0	3·0	3·0	5·0	3·0	2·0	3·0
Infant deaths before discharge per 1000 live births*	2·43	2·18	7·35	14·91	12·83	30·96	13·74	9·85	27·93	11·96	11·87	12·08
Total fetal/neonatal death rate per 1000 total births*†	15·34	15·01	21·58	32·55	27·28	71·56	29·02	26·21	39·11	21·40	23·96	17·80

* These figures, being based upon differing periods of exposure to risk, are not comparable and should be interpreted with caution
† Includes fetal/neonatal deaths where time of death was unknown (which were excluded in the stillbirth and neonatal death rates)

patients at this facility. In Honduras, the large maternity hospital is supported by the Ministry of Health. Since there is no charge to the patients, the clientele consists of the indigent; those with medical coverage obtain care at a social security or private hospital. In Venezuela, the large general teaching hospital is essentially supported by the Ministry of Health, so that patients do not pay for their care.

AGE AND PARITY

The age distributions are similar in the four hospitals with approximately 80% of patients less than 30 years old in each hospital. The percentage of women who have not had a previous delivery is higher in Santiago and Campinas – over 35% – than in Tegucigalpa and Cumaná – 30% or less. Figure 1 gives the number of deliveries and proportion of cesareans by age and parity (parity equals live births plus stillbirths, present delivery *not* included) in each of the four hospitals. For each of the parity levels, the percentage of cesareans is higher for older than for younger women in all the hospitals, though the difference is small for grand multiparas in Campinas. Distinctions are most pronounced for nulliparous women, the older patients having cesarean rates 20–30 percentage points above those of the younger.

The Mantel–Haenszel[1] procedure is used to test whether, on the average, across hospital and parity levels, the rates of cesarean delivery are the same for the two age groups or are consistently different. This statistic is compared to the χ^2 distribution, with appropriate degrees of freedom, to determine statistical significance. Controlling for each of the parity levels in the four hospitals, the Mantel–Haenszel statistic is highly significant ($p < 0.01$). Furthermore, with the exception of the highest parity level in Campinas, older women have a significantly larger proportion of cesareans at each parity level in each hospital ($p < 0.05$).

Figure 1 also shows that the percentage of cesarean deliveries decreases with increasing parity in each age group of each hospital. Controlling for the two age levels in the four hospitals, the Mantel–Haenszel statistic is highly significant ($p < 0.01$). Additionally, statistically significant inverse associations between percentage of cesareans and parity level were found in each of the eight subpopulations defined by hospital location and age level ($p < 0.05$).

In all four hospitals, the women with the highest rate of cesareans are

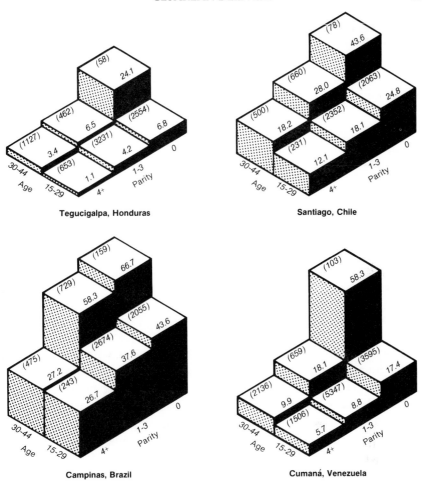

Tegucigalpa, Honduras

Santiago, Chile

Campinas, Brazil

Cumaná, Venezuela

Figure 1   Cesarean delivery by parity and age at four Latin American hospitals

primiparas over 30 years of age and the lowest rate is for grand multiparas 15–20 years old. Thus, while cesarean rates vary widely between hospitals, within each hospital the same pattern with respect to age and parity holds.

INDICATIONS FOR CESAREAN DELIVERY

In this section, differential rates of cesarean birth are investigated with respect to different indications for cesareans, and by the likelihood of performing a cesarean, given any indication. The implications of these

Table 3 Percentage of women with indication for cesarean delivery by type of indication, for women with no previous deliveries

Indication	Tegucigalpa, Honduras (%)	Cumaná, Venezuela (%)	Santiago, Chile (%)	Campinas, Brazil (%)
Fetal	14·3	32·1	52·2	59·5
CPD	0·0	0·6	8·7	11·4
Obstructed labor	6·4	12·2	7·2	20·3
Prolonged labor	1·0	5·5	4·7	1·2
Fetal distress	4·3	3·5	8·9	11·0
Other*	2·6	10·2	22·7	15·6
Maternal†	2·7	13·7	7·2	13·4
No recorded indication	83·0	54·2	40·6	27·1
n =	2559	3645	2083	2181

* Includes breech, other malpresentations, cord prolapse and failed induction
† Includes placenta previa, placenta abruptio, toxemia, diabetes, hypertensive disorders, renal disorders, hyper- and hypo-uterine contractions and primipara ⩾ 35 years of age.
  Note: Total is 100%. Women designated as having a more severe indication are coded as having that indication and not for lesser indications

two factors for variations in hospital cesarean rates are explored in Tables 3 and 4. This analysis is confined to women who are having their first delivery. The usual practice of examining indications for surgical delivery among women with no history of cesareans is not followed here. This is because parous women, with a proven ability to deliver vaginally, are less likely to have indications for cesareans in subsequent deliveries than are nulliparous women. Confining the discussion to the latter category eliminates the confounding influence of parity in affecting the indications for a cesarean.

Deliveries are categorized by whether there is a recorded indication for a cesarean. If there is an indication recorded, it is further classified as either fetal or maternal. The fetal indications are subclassified as cephalopelvic disproportion, obstructed labor, prolonged labor, fetal distress or other. The category 'other' includes breech and other malpresentations, cord prolapse and failed induction of labor. Maternal indications included are placenta previa, placenta abruptio, toxemia, diabetes, hypertensive disorders, renal disorders, hyper- and hypo-uterine contractions and primipara ≥35 years of age.

The most striking difference among these hospitals is in the proportion of women with no recorded indication for cesareans (among all women regardless of type of delivery), from a high of 83%

in Tegucigalpa to a low of 27% in Campinas. The same pattern occurs with respect to fetal and maternal indications, except that in Santiago the percentage with maternal indications is lower than in Cumaná. Specifically, in Honduras cephalopelvic disproportion (CDP) is never reported, is less than 1% in Cumaná, but 9% in Santiago and 11% in Campinas. The proportion of women with obstructed labor also follows a similar pattern, except that it is higher in Cumaná than in

Table 4 Percentage of women delivering by cesarean, by type of indication, for women with no previous deliveries

Indication	Tegucigalpa, Honduras		Cumaná, Venezuela		Santiago, Chile		Campinas, Brazil	
	%	No.	%	No.	%	No.	%	No.
Fetal	45·4	366	37·0	1169	47·2	1088	64·6	1293
CPD	—	0	95·7	23	90·6	181	99·2	248
Obstructed labor	89·0	164	36·2	445	44·4	151	81·2	442
Prolonged labor	11·5	26	26·9	201	35·7	98	53·8	26
Fetal distress	1·8	109	38·5	129	51·1	186	61·0	241
Other*	22·4	67	39·6	371	32·4	472	21·4	341
Maternal†	10·0	70	21·6	501	9·3	150	20·5	292
No recorded indication	0·1	2123	6·4	1975	0·5	845	14·9	591

* Includes breech, other malpresentations, cord prolapse and failed induction.
† Includes placenta previa, placenta abruptio, toxemia, diabetes, hypertensive disorders, renal disorders, hyper- and hypo-uterine contractions and primipara $\nmid$ 35 years of age.

Santiago. When these two categories are combined, as they often are, the pattern is again one of a rising rate, moving from the Honduran to the Brazilian hospital. The proportion with fetal distress also follows this pattern, though with irregularities.

Table 4 shows the percentages of cesareans performed by indication for abdominal delivery. Not only is this proportion (45%) significantly higher in Campinas than elsewhere ($p < 0·01$), but so, too, is the proportion (15%) of women who have cesareans with no reported indication ($p < 0·01$). The rate for maternal indications is significantly lower than that for the fetus in each of the hospitals ($p < 0·01$).

As displayed by Figure 2, the proportion of women with reported indications for cesareans increases significantly ($p < 0·01$) with the rate of surgery. It is unlikely that the real range of indications could be as

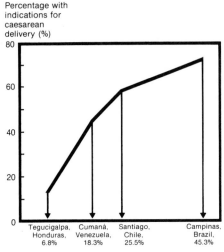

Figure 2 Indication for cesarean delivery for primiparas at four Latin American hospitals

wide as is reported; rather, it may be the likelihood of reporting an indication that varies with cesarean rates. We will return to this hypothesis later.

EMERGENCY VERSUS ELECTIVE CESAREAN DELIVERY

Data on the indication for the cesarean are limited, so the investigator must resort to other indicators to determine the circumstances influencing the decisions. Variations in the frequency of blood transfusions, the choice of anesthetic and differences in nights hospitalized according to the type of delivery are considered.

A blood transfusion suggests an emergency operation. Among the mothers undergoing surgery in Tegucigalpa, 23% received a blood transfusion compared with 4·4% in Cumaná, 10% in Santiago and 3·5% in Campinas. The higher percentage requiring transfusions in the Honduran hospital suggests that emergency patients may make up a much higher percentage of cesareans there than in the other three hospitals.

Figure 3 shows that the percentage of patients with cesarean deliveries who receive a general anesthetic decreases as the cesarean

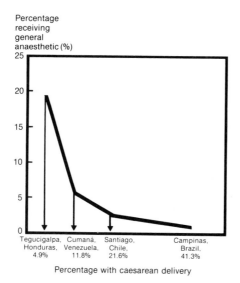

Figure 3   General anesthesia and cesarean delivery at four Latin American hospitals

rate increases. Further, in the Honduran hospital, the proportion given a general anesthetic is significantly higher ($p<0\cdot05$) among primary than repeat cesarean patients (25% *vs* 9%). The greater use of general anesthetics in Honduras is a reflection of the emergency character of the cesareans. In general, anesthesiologists prefer spinal anesthetics but use general anesthetics in emergencies, especially those involving hemorrhages with some type of shock. Thus among all cesarean births, their use would be expected to be greater the higher the proportion of emergencies, and indeed a greater proportion of primary, as compared to repeat, cesareans are expected to be emergencies.

In the three hospitals with higher rates of abdominal delivery, the similarity in use of anesthetics among primary and repeat cases indicates similar treatment of the two groups of patients; suggesting that emergency cases do not constitute the preponderance of cesarean deliveries. The percentage of women receiving general anesthetics for primary and repeat cesarean deliveries at the three hospitals is as follows: Cumaná ($6\cdot4\%$, $6\cdot8\%$), Santiago ($3\cdot8\%$, $2\cdot8\%$), Campinas ($0\cdot2\%$, $0\cdot0\%$).

Perhaps the best overall indication of the relative contribution of emergency cesareans to the total of cesareans is found in the differences in median nights hospitalized between women delivered by cesarean and those delivered vaginally. The difference estimates the additional contribution that cesarean delivery makes to length of hospital stay. As shown in Figure 4, the difference in the median values of cesarean and vaginal postdelivery hospitalization decreases as the rate of cesareans increases. This, too, provides indirect evidence that cesarean patients in hospitals with low cesarean delivery rates required emergency care whereas those in hospitals with higher rates generally did not. In Honduras, where women are rarely hospitalized for more than one night for regular delivery, the long stay of cesarean patients (median stay is 5·3 nights) is a strong indication of the medical problems that necessitated it. In contrast, it may be inferred from the small difference in Campinas that many cesareans are elective.

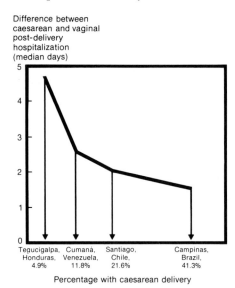

Figure 4   Differential maternal postpartum hospitalization and cesarean delivery at four Latin American hospitals

   Although the proportion of women having medical indications for a cesarean increases with its rate, the proportion of cesareans that are emergency cases (using the indicator difference in median nights hospitalized between women delivered vaginally and abdominally) decreases significantly with the rate of cesareans ($p < 0·05$). Therefore, reported medical indications for this surgery by hospital may be of limited use in explaining the wide variation in the rates. Although every cesarean is indicated in the eyes of the physician performing it, variations in practices of reporting those indications may be so great as to make these data of little use in arriving at an understanding of the cause of such a great diversity in cesarean rates.

COSTS OF CESAREAN VERSUS VAGINAL DELIVERIES

The extra cost of performing a cesarean compared with a vaginal delivery may be assessed by calculating the extra resources entailed in the surgery. The total savings would, of course, be greater the higher the cesarean rate. Therefore, the reductions could be greater in Campinas than in the other hospitals.

These calculations are based on the assumption that the average patient having a cesarean delivery is the same at all four hospitals. In practice, as we have argued in the preceding section, women delivered abdominally in Tegucigalpa are more likely to be emergency patients than in Campinas. Consequently, if the cesarean rate in Tegucigalpa were to be reduced, costs might even increase. For example, if among those cases in which a cesarean is performed to stop hemorrhaging and save the lives of the mother and the fetus, a vaginal delivery were to be performed, not only would the survival chances of the mother and child be compromised, but also, additional blood loss might lead to an increase in blood administered. With this caveat in mind, we assess the following resource savings:

(1) anesthetics
(2) blood transfusions
(3) nights hospitalized
(4) attendants at delivery

For the four hospitals, the difference in the percentage of women receiving anesthetics by type of delivery decreases as the percentage of women having a cesarean increases. It appears that hospitals that intervene by performing cesareans also intervene by administering anesthetics to women delivering vaginally. In Campinas, only 18% of these non-surgical patients receive no anesthetic as compared with 33% in Santiago and over 50% of the same groups in Cumaná and Tegucigalpa. As a consequence of its greater use during vaginal deliveries in hospitals with high cesarean rates, the cost savings of decreasing the number of cesareans are diminished.

The cost savings with respect to reducing blood transfusions and nights hospitalized are also less in hospitals with higher cesarean rates, because their average cesarean patient neither spends much more time in hospital nor is very much more likely to receive a blood transfusion than is the woman with a vaginal delivery. But, as discussed earlier, it is probably only in the hospitals with the higher cesarean rates that the cost savings can be realized without endangering the life of the mother and/or child.

In almost every case, an obstetrician or gynecologist is the primary attendant at a cesarean birth. In contrast, many vaginal deliveries in Tegucigalpa and Campinas are attended by medical students, so that cost savings will vary, depending on who is in attendance.

Paradoxically, we then find, in considering the average patient, both vaginal and cesarean, that eliminating 'excess' cesarean deliveries has little impact on cost savings per patient in hospitals that perform fewer cesareans because hospitals with a high rate tend to intervene in many ways (e.g. use of anesthetic and the attendance of an obstetrician/gynecologist at vaginal delivery). In hospitals with low rates, the calculated potential cost savings are not borne out in practice. Women with cesareans have more medical problems than the other mothers. Consequently, reductions in cesareans may be costly in terms of lives, and perhaps, also, of resources. If we could compare similar women, we would have a better picture of cost savings. But the data on indications are not reliable enough to 'select' women with similar medical indications for surgical delivery.

Data collected by the FHI show a wide variation in rates of cesarean delivery in 20 Latin American hospitals from a low of $2\cdot8\%$ in a Honduran hospital to a high of $49\cdot1\%$ in a Brazilian one.

The role of socio-demographic and medical factors in affecting variations in cesarean rates has been explored for four of these hospitals. With respect to age and parity, these rates were highest among older women with first deliveries in each of the four hospitals.

Although the percentage of women with medical indications for cesarean increases with the cesarean rate, other data suggest that documented medical indications are of limited value in explaining variations in these rates. The proportion that may be classified as emergency decreases with the cesarean rate. Hospitals that do not customarily perform this surgery may be reluctant or simply unaccustomed to classifying women as having indications for cesarean unless there are grounds for believing that the mother and/or child would be jeopardized by a vaginal birth. In hospitals with higher rates, the operation is more routinely practiced and physicians may classify more women as having medical indications for surgical deliveries.

Even though the data suggest that costs could be reduced if the cesarean rate fell, these findings are somewhat illusory. Where cesareans are not a matter of routine, these patients are expensive emergencies, but hospitals in which cesareans are common practice are geared to special care of their patients. Consequently, the vaginally delivered patient is also carefully attended.

The feasibility of reducing cesarean deliveries at hospitals with low rates is open to question. In fact, it may be argued that additional resources should be devoted to increasing the number of cesareans at the Honduran hospital. In Campinas, however, some cost savings might be realized without endangering the health of mother or child.

References

1 Mantel, N. and Haenszel, W. (1959). Statistical aspects of the analysis of data from retrospective studies of disease. *J. Natl. Cancer Inst.*, **22**, 719
2 Placek, P.J. and Taffel, S.M. (1980). Trends in cesarean section rates for the United States, 1970–78. *Public Health Rep.*, **85**(6), 540
3 Rosen, M.G. (1981). NIH consensus development task force statement on cesarean childbirth. *Am. J. Obstet. Gynecol.*, **139**, 902

5

Deliveries after cesarean birth in two Asian university hospitals

I. CHI, A. B. SAIFUDDIN, D. E. GUNATILAKE and S. L. WALLACE

One of the significant recommendations made by the task force of the consensus conference on cesarean birth, sponsored by the National Institutes of Health (NIH), for curbing the ever-increasing cesarean birthrate in the United States was to substitute routine elective repeat cesarean delivery with a trial of labor and subsequent vaginal delivery in adequately selected cases[6]. Because more than 98% of US women with a previous cesarean delivery undergo a repeat cesarean for subsequent pregnancies[6], and the number of women delivered vaginally after previous cesarean birth in a hospital is generally too small for comparison with the former[1], we used data from two Asian teaching hospitals to assess the benefits and risks associated with this recommendation.

The two Asian medical centers studied were the General Hospital, University of Indonesia, Jakarta, Indonesia, and the De Soysa Hospital for Women, Colombo, Sri Lanka. They were chosen because the medical care systems differed in each country; basically, fee for services in the former and socialized health care in the latter.

In the Jakarta General Hospital, records were collected for 106 women who had previously been delivered by cesarean and were admitted for a subsequent delivery between January and November 1978. All the deliveries were singletons. Among them, 63 (59·4%) were delivered vaginally and the remaining 43 by repeat cesarean. (Among the latter, four had two previous cesarean deliveries.) As shown in the two left columns of Table 1, mean age was nearly identical between the vaginal delivery and repeat cesarean groups. More women in the latter group were primiparas prior to this pregnancy (therefore their only previous birth was delivered abdominally). However, the proportion of women having one or more antenatal visits before this delivery was higher in the former group ($\chi^2 = 6 \cdot 19$, $p < 0 \cdot 05$). The fact that more than half of the women in both groups were delivered on the day of admission suggests that the majority of them were admitted after labor started. Also, only about one fifth of the repeat cesarean group was delivered with no labor, and more than 90% of them had some complications of labor and/or delivery. This seems to indicate that most of the repeat cesareans in this

Table 1 Selected information on index delivery subsequent to previous cesarean delivery by method of delivery for the General Hospital, University of Indonesia, Jakarta, Indonesia, and De Soysa Hospital for Women, Colombo, Sri Lanka, 1977–1978

	Jakarta hospital		Colombo hospital	
	Vaginal delivery	Repeat cesarean	Vaginal delivery	Repeat cesarean
No. of women	63	43	30	121
No. of infants delivered	63	43	32	122
Mean age in years	27·6	28·0	31·6	31·3
% Primipara (prior to this delivery)	34·9	44·2	76·7	66·9
% With one or more antenatal visits	85·7	65·1	100·0	98·3
% Delivered same day as admission	55·7	62·8	20·0	9·2
% Delivered with no labor	0·0	23·3	0·0	92·5
% With some complications during labor/delivery	18·0	90·7	10·0	6·6
% Maternal deaths	0·0	2·3	0·0	0·0
% Stillbirths	1·6	2·3	6·7	0·8
% Neonatal deaths	0·0	7·1	6·7	3·3
% Blood transfusion	1·6	46·5	3·3	4·1
% Febrile morbidity	0·0	4·7	0·0	7·4
% Premature infants ($< 2500\,\mathrm{g}$)	9·8	9·3	39·3*	20·8*
% Sterilization performed before discharge	23·8	45·2	6·7	43·0
% Hospitalized eight or more nights after delivery	1·6	95·3	16·7	99·2

* Singleton deliveries only. If prematurity is defined as $\langle 2250\,\mathrm{g}$, the proportions of premature infants will be 21·4% for the vaginal delivery group and 6·7% for the repeat cesarean group

hospital were performed for some medical indication rather than based on the 'once a cesarean, always a cesarean' doctrine. Some women were probably delivered on an emergency basis immediately upon arrival[2], hence, the remarkably high blood transfusion rate in this group.

In the vaginal group, there was one stillbirth, a case of poly-hydramnios. In the repeat cesarean group, there was one maternal death, one stillbirth and three neonatal deaths. The maternal death occurred in a 22-year-old, para 2 woman who arrived in the hospital in the first stage of labor with a diagnosis of cephalopelvic disproportion. The cesarean was performed under general anesthesia. She died of aspiration pneumonia soon after delivery; the infant survived. The stillbirth occurred in a fetus as a result of neglected transverse lie; the mother suffered a uterine rupture and had a laparotomy upon admission. She survived and was discharged about a week after delivery. As for the three neonatal deaths, one occurred in a low-birth-weight (1700 g) baby delivered of a 23-year-old, para 6 woman at a gestational age of 30 weeks; only one of her previous six births had survived. Another neonatal death was a 3050 g frank breech infant suffering from stress during labor. Intrapartum infection and fetal distress were mentioned on the record for the third death. Three of the four perinatal deaths could probably have been avoided, had the patients been admitted to the hospital earlier.

Of the total cases studied, five patients (4·7%) suffered uterine rupture. In one case, the baby was delivered vaginally, assisted by outlet forceps. The other four ended in repeat cesarean delivery; all mothers and three of the four infants involved were discharged alive, and the one stillbirth has been discussed above. In this hospital, all deliveries for women with previous cesarean delivery were attended by physicians, mostly obstetricians.

Between January 1977 and June 1978, records were collected for 151 women with previous cesarean delivery(ies) who were admitted to the Colombo Hospital for subsequent delivery. As shown in the two right columns of Table 1, 30 (19·9%) of them were delivered vaginally and the remaining 121 by repeat cesarean. One patient in the former and 21 in the latter group had two previous cesarean deliveries (one woman had three previous deliveries). Women in the two delivery groups were of almost identical mean age, but the proportion of primiparas (prior to this delivery) was slightly higher in the vaginal group than in the repeat cesarean group. The Sri Lanka women displayed a very different picture in their antepartum conditions compared to their Indonesian counterparts, probably because of their socialized health care system. Irrespective of the delivery methods, nearly all women had one or more antenatal visit. The majority of women in both groups were admitted at least one day before delivery (hence most before active labor had started), and very few had any labor/delivery complications. The fact that over 90% of the women in the repeat cesarean group did not experience labor suggests that many of these repeat sections were done on an elective basis, primarily because of the previous cesarean delivery. The low blood transfusion rate in this group supports this deduction. The proportion of low-birth-weight (<2500 g) babies was lower in the repeat cesarean group than in the vaginal group ($\chi^2=4\cdot20$, $p<0\cdot05$), suggesting that iatrogenic prematurity was not a major problem.

There were no maternal deaths in either group. Two stillbirths and two neonatal deaths occurred in the vaginal group, and one stillbirth and four neonatal deaths occurred in the repeat cesarean group. Excluding the two sets of twins delivered in the vaginal group and one set in the repeat cesarean group, this gives an uncorrected perinatal mortality of $107\cdot1$ (per 1000 infants delivered) for the former group and $42\cdot0$ for the latter group. This difference is based on small numbers and is not statistically significant ($p=0\cdot18$ by Fisher's exact test). Three of the four perinatal deaths in the vaginal group were under 2000 g (one of the deaths occurred in a twin delivery with a birth weight of 1580 g), while none of the five perinatal deaths in the repeat cesarean group weighed less than 2000 g. No uterine ruptures were reported for either group.

As also shown in Table 1, in both hospitals, the proportion of women undergoing concurrent tubal sterilization was consistently higher in the repeat cesarean than in the vaginal group (p values $<0\cdot01$ by χ^2 test), suggesting that some of the sterilizations in the former group might not have been performed if the abdominal approach had not been taken.

In both hospitals, febrile morbidity was only reported for women in the repeat cesarean group. This finding cannot be attributed to the higher tubal sterilization rate in the repeat section group. The two patients reporting fever in the Jakarta Hospital did not have a concurrent sterilization. For the nine patients reporting fever from the Colombo Hospital, five did not have a sterilization.

The most apparent and consistent finding for the two hospitals was

Table 2 Mean no. of nights hospitalized after index delivery by tubal sterilization status and method of delivery for the General Hospital, University of Indonesia, Jakarta, Indonesia, and De Soysa Hospital for Women, Colombo, Sri Lanka, 1977–1978[a]

Concurrent tubal sterilization	Method of delivery	Jakarta hospital			Colombo hospital		
		No. of women	Mean no. of nights	p values[b]	No. of women[c]	Mean no. of nights	p values[b]
No	Vaginal delivery	48	3·6	< 0·01	28	3·3	< 0·01
	Repeat cesarean	24	7·9		68	8·0	
Yes	Vaginal delivery	15	4·6	< 0·01	2	6·5	< 0·07
	Repeat cesarean	19	7·8		52	8·0	

[a] On the Maternity Record, women who stayed for more than eight nights were recorded as if they stayed for exactly eight nights
[b] By Fisher's exact test
[c] The sterilization status was unknown for one woman at the Colombo Hospital

in the length of hospitalization following delivery. While over 80% of the women in the vaginal group in both hospitals were discharged within 5 days, rarely was a woman in the repeat cesarean group discharged less than 8 days after delivery (p values $< 0 \cdot 001$ by Fisher's exact test). The greater proportion of patients having concurrent tubal sterilization in the repeat cesarean group cannot explain this difference. Hospitalization was consistently longer for the repeat cesarean patients than the vaginal group in both hospitals for those who had a concurrent sterilization as well as for those who did not. The differences were more marked in women with no concurrent sterilization. Table 2 illustrates the magnitude as well as the statistical significance of the differences.

Electronic fetal monitoring devices were not available during the study period at either hospital. Oxytocin was rarely used in the vaginal delivery group. Information on hysterectomy was only available for one patient who had a uterine rupture in the Jakarta Hospital. Identical proportions (26·7%) of the vaginal deliveries in the two hospitals were assisted by forceps or vacuum extraction.

Finally, a word about patients with more than one previous cesarean. In the Colombo Hospital, the one woman who had had two previous cesarean deliveries and who was delivered vaginally for the current birth fared well. The 21 women with more than one previous cesarean delivery in the repeat cesarean group contributed two of the four neonatal deaths mentioned above. They also had a higher puerperal complication rate than women who had only one previous section. However, this difference is not statistically significant, and the complications were minor in nature, mostly wound infections.

No information was available from the Maternity Record on (a) whether multiparous women were delivered vaginally before or after the previous cesarean birth, (b) the indications for and complications of the previous cesareans, and (c) indications for the repeat cesareans at this admission. The general condition of the women upon arrival at the hospitals for the current delivery was also not recorded. Thus, it is difficult to judge whether the decision made on the method of delivery was justified. Also, because the causes of perinatal deaths were not sufficiently described, it is difficult to judge whether some of these deaths could have been avoided, had the alternative delivery method been employed. The most important information on the type of previous cesarean was also not recorded, but we know in actuality that most, if not all, the procedures were of the low cervical transverse type. Finally, no information was available on the proportion of women who were switched to repeat cesarean delivery after failure of trial of labor, so we were forced to classify the women by performed method rather than intended method of delivery.

Despite the limited information, it is apparent that the nature of patients undergoing repeat cesarean is different between the two hospitals. For the Jakarta hospital, it seems that a considerable proportion of patients who had had a previous cesarean had been subjected to a kind of natural experiment for trial of labor before their admission to the hospital. Thus, most of repeat cesareans after admission could be considered as the consequence of a failure in trial of labor. In this sense, the fact that about 60% of the patients had a vaginal delivery at this admission is particularly significant; this proportion probably approximates the extent of possible vaginal delivery following a previous cesarean delivery and is generally in keeping with the results from the few reports in the US[3,5] and Britain[4]. Also, the total maternal and infant mortality and morbidity would probably approximate what would happen when a group of women with previous cesarean delivery were subjected to trial of labor.

On the other hand, the repeat cesareans performed in the Colombo hospital seemed to be performed mostly on an elective basis, probably most of them a result of the 'once a cesarean, always a cesarean' dictum and a few because of an intended tubal sterilization. The number of switchovers from failure of trial of labor is probably negligible and, hence, comparisons between the two delivery groups are more justified. Ostensibly, 'perinatal' mortality was higher in the vaginal delivery group than in the repeat cesarean group, but this may have been due to a policy of allowing stillbirths and small premature infants to be delivered vaginally. The much shorter hospital stay of patients in the vaginal group coupled with the fact that more than half of them (53·3%) were delivered by trained midwives (all repeat cesarean procedures were performed by obstetricians) signify the considerable savings of medical costs for vaginal delivery subsequent to primary cesarean delivery in adequately chosen women.

The remarkably longer hospital stay for the repeat cesarean group in both hospitals may lead us to a misinterpretation of morbidity and mortality data because of the longer observational period, hence a greater chance of detecting such morbidity and mortality in the former group. While this might be true for morbidity such as fever, it can be argued the other way around that some maternal morbidity not included in the comparison must be considerably higher in the repeat cesarean group, which was actually the reason for their longer hospital stay. As for the mortality data, this concern may not be justified, as all mothers and newborns were in satisfactory condition when discharged from the hospital. It is unlikely that deaths would occur in significant numbers in the vaginal delivery group in the few days following their discharge at which time their counterparts in the repeat cesarean group were also discharged.

Findings from these two Asian hospitals, in general, support the recommendation made by the NIH task force in that (a) for a considerable proportion of women with previous cesarean delivery, their subsequent pregnancy can be delivered vaginally with no significantly increased maternal and infant mortality and morbidity, and (b) the savings in medical cost for the vaginal deliveries after previous cesarean delivery are considerable as compared to the repeat cesareans. However, more studies from developing countries specially designed for clarifying this issue are needed.

References

1 Bottom, S. E., Rosen, M. G. and Sokol, R. J. (1980). The increase in cesarean birth rate. *N. Engl. J. Med.*, **302**, 559

2 Chi, I-c., Agoestina, T. and Harbin, J. (1981). Maternal mortality at twelve teaching hospitals in Indonesia – an epidemiologic analysis. *Int. J. Gynaecol Obstet.*, **19**, 259

3 Douglas, R. G., Birnbaum, S. J. and MacDonald, F. A. (1963). Pregnancy and labor following cesarean section. *Am. J. Obstet. Gynecol.*, **86**, 961

4 McGarry, J. A. (1969). The management of patients previously delivered by cesarean section. *J. Obstet. Gynaecol. Br. Commonw.*, **76**, 137

5 Merrill, B. S. and Gibbs, C. E. (1978). Planned vaginal delivery following cesarean sections. *Obstet. Gynecol.*, **52**, 50

6 Rosen, M. G. (1981). NIH consensus development task force statement on cesarean childbirth. *Am. J. Obstet. Gynecol.*, **139**, 902

6

Management of breech presentations: vaginal or abdominal delivery?

J. A. FORTNEY, K. I. KENNEDY and L. E. LAUFE

Infants presenting in the breech position are jeopardized for a number of reasons. Breech babies are more likely than other babies to have major congenital anomalies, especially at the earlier gestations[4,8,12,16]; they are more likely to be of low birth weight[4,7,18]; they are more likely to involve multiple gestations; and their delivery is more likely to be associated with additional complications (such as cord prolapse) than the deliveries of other infants[11,13,15]. In addition, delivery itself poses a greater hazard to breech babies than to babies presenting by vertex. Since this last factor is the only one that the attending physican can influence, it has received a fair amount of attention. While few authors recommend cesarean delivery routinely for all breech infants, many recommend expansion of the indications for cesarean[2,3,11]. For some time, cesarean delivery was not recommended for premature breeches; as recently as 1967, external version (repeatedly if necessary) and vaginal delivery were being recommended for all but footling premature breeches[11]. More recently, however, most authors have recommended abdominal delivery for the small breech infant[8,9,12,15,19,20] as well as for the very large[21]. Exceptions are Bowes et al.[2] who found no significant difference by delivery technique in the survival of 151 infants weighing 501 to 2500 g, and both Cruikshank and Pitkin[7] and Lewis and Seneviratne[17] who argue strongly that the case has not yet been made for routine abdominal delivery of the low-birth-weight breech baby. The NIH Cesarean Birth Task Force concluded that the data were insufficient to make a firm recommendation on method of delivery of the low-birth-weight breech baby[24].

In a symposium sponsored by the journal *Contemporary Ob/Gyn* on the management of breeches, the participants concluded that the physician's experience was a crucial factor, and that the inexperienced physician should always deliver abdominally, although more experienced obstetricians could successfully deliver vaginally[5]. Karp and colleagues[15] recommend trial of labor for premature breeches except in the case of footling breech or when there are any other complications. At least one recent article[17] contends that with continuous fetal monitoring, vaginal delivery is preferred unless there are additional complications.

Cesarean delivery is unique among surgical procedures in that it involves risk to two patients. Furthermore, it can be performed either for fetal or maternal reasons. In the case of breech presentations, fetal reasons predominate. Cesarean surgery, however, carries risk for future childbearing. The physician must choose the means to deliver a fetus he knows to be of questionable viability simply by the fact that it is breech; the safest means for the mother, i.e. vaginal, may produce a stillborn infant or a severely compromised infant with potentially permanent damage. The safest means for the infant, i.e. abdominal, may also produce a stillborn or compromised infant, and furthermore threaten the mother's life and future reproductive health. Hibbard[14] reports a large increase in the number of surgically delivered infants with lethal defects in 1974 compared with 1965 when the use of cesarean delivery was less liberal.

Bowes *et al.*[2] report an increase in maternal morbidity from 7% to 15% as the section rate for breeches increased from 13% to 54%. Collea and his colleagues[6] found 49% morbidity among mothers delivered abdominally compared with only 7% among mothers delivered vaginally, and 2 of the 140 mothers delivered abdominally required hysterectomies – a serious consequence for any parturient, but especially for the mother of a potentially compromised baby. Collea's work is particularly important because it reports the only study of the management of (term) breeches that involved a randomized trial. Petitti and colleagues[22], using data from births in California for the years 1973–1975, found a maternal mortality rate for cesarean births that was twice that for vaginal births; Evrard and Gold[10] found that the risk of death from cesarean delivery was 26 times higher than for vaginal delivery in Rhode Island from 1965 to 1975. Recent work from the Center for Disease Control[26] shows deaths from cesarean surgery to be significantly underreported, at least in Georgia. By matching death certificates of women aged 10–44 with live birth certificates for a similar time period, Rubin and his colleagues found that the total death-to-case rate is 105·3 deaths per 100 000 cesarean sections, and that 59·3 of these can be attributed to the cesarean surgery alone (i.e. and not to the conditions for which it was performed).

Thus, although some authors state that, for example, 'perinatal morbidity can be reduced at no significant cost in terms of maternal morbidity[19], others recognize that 'the maternal side of the perennial obstetric equation' remains largely unknown[25].

Much of the research on the management of the breech presentation suffers from one or more defects in either design or analysis. For example, although most studies exclude multiple gestations, very few exclude either antepartum deaths or congenital anomalies; Bowes[2] is an exception to this.

The overriding problem in research into this problem is that of sample size. All studies published to date suffer from the small number of cases available for analysis, and this is especially true of studies of the low-birth-weight breech. The small numbers mean that analysis is severely restricted; it becomes impossible, for instance, to compare the outcome of different methods of delivery for the different types of breech in different weight categories. Even in the large data set available to us, of the 157 cases of footling infants weighing less than 1500 g, only 11 were delivered by cesarean.

It is obviously difficult to find a large number of cases of any rare event, and only about 4% of deliveries involve a breech presentation. Therefore, studies of breech presentations sometimes involve deliveries occurring over a period of several years; Goldenberg and Nelson's[12] cases were spread over 5 years, Galloway's[11] over 11 years. This poses a problem for the interpretation of the data, not only because the management of breech has changed in recent years, but more importantly because the resources to manage the high-risk infant have improved enormously over the past several years. Since the trend toward increased use of cesarean delivery occurred simultaneously with increased chances of the infant surviving because of improved resources, it is difficult to separate the two effects.

Another possibility is to combine the data from many hospitals to obtain sufficient numbers for analysis. The problems here are similar to those of combining data over time – different hospitals have different resources, physicians of different levels of skill and patients in different risk categories. The design of the research proposed here is intended specifically to overcome this problem.

There were almost 17000 breech presentations in the pool of Maternity Records from all contributing centers. From these we eliminated (1) multiple gestations, (2) antepartum deaths and (3) congenital anomalies. These were excluded for theoretical reasons. For practical reasons we also excluded (4) some hospitals and some individual cases where we considered there to be problems of data quality, (5) hospitals with fewer than 25 cases of breech presentations (after exclusions 1–3 were made). After these exclusions there remained 11524 cases or 68% of the original pool. These cases came from 90 hospitals widely distributed around the world.

The 90 hospitals were then divided into three categories of similar size according to the level of mortality (before maternal hospital discharge) of *all* babies (i.e. not only the breech babies) delivered in the hospital. All hospitals with a 'perinatal' mortality level of 45 per 1000 deliveries or higher were categorized as high mortality and averaged 82·5 per 1000 deliveries. Hospitals with a 'perinatal' mortality rate between 20·9 and 44·9 per 1000 deliveries for all babies were categorized as having medium mortality, and these averaged a mortality rate of 30·9 per 1000. Low mortality hospitals were defined as having a mortality rate before maternal discharge of less than 20·9 per 1000, and they averaged 15·1 per 1000. The cutpoints are arbitrary and are designed primarily to produce groups of similar size.

The three mortality categories reflect not only the skills of the physicians and midwives attending deliveries, but also the hospital facilities and resources, the kinds of patients admitted, whether the hospital is a referral hospital with a large percentage of high-risk patients, or a hospital that refers its high-risk patients elsewhere, and even the average duration of postpartum hospital stay. Unfortunately, for the most part, we know almost nothing about the facilities available, especially the availability of pediatricians or perinatologists. Furthermore, while it would be desirable to separate these various factors, they did not prove to be readily quantifiable and separable. The location and type of hospitals in the three categories are shown in Table 1.

Because of the interrelationships among the factors that contribute to the overall perinatal mortality rate, the distribution of these factors is shown in Tables 2–5. Table 2 shows that the mortality of the breech births before the mothers' discharges from the hospital was 3·5 times

Table 1 Contributing hospitals by mortality categories

	High	Medium	Low
General hospitals			
Brazil			1
El Salvador			1
Taiwan			1
Chile		1	
Panama		1	
Tanzania		1	
Egypt	1	1	
India	1	2	
Bangladesh	1		
Maternity hospitals			
Bangladesh			1
Peru			1
W. Germany			1
Iran		1	
Mali		1	
Senegal		1	
Sri Lanka		1	
Rwanda	1		
Private clinics			
Bangladesh			1
India		1	1
Multicenter studies			
Colombia		2	2
Classification uncertain			
Belgium			1
Italy		1	1
Teaching hospitals			
Austria			1
Ireland			1
Italy			2
Japan			1
Malta			1
Mexico			1
Scotland			1
Singapore			1
Sweden			1
Thailand			2
Venezuela			1
W. Germany			2
Brazil	3		1

Table 1 (cont'd)

	High	Medium	Low
Egypt	4		1
Pakistan	1		1
Canada		1	
Chile		3	
Costa Rica		1	
El Salvador		1	
Hungary		2	
Sierra Leone		1	
Sri Lanka		1	
Yugoslavia		1	
India	3	1	
Indonesia	1	3	
Bangladesh	13		
Nigeria	1		
Peru	1		
Total	31	29	30

Table 2 Characteristics of the three strata

	High	Medium	Low
No. of breeches delivered	3921	3988	3615
No. of centers	31	29	30
Perinatal mortality rate for *all* babies in these centers	82·5	30·9	15·1
Perinatal mortality rate for *breech* babies in these centers	114·0	54·9	32·3
No. of maternal deaths	14	5	1
Maternal death rate (per 1000 deliveries)	3·6	1·3	0·3

higher in the high mortality hospitals than in the low mortality hospitals. (This refers only to singleton breeches, alive at the onset of labor and with no congenital malformations; had these exclusions not been made, the mortality would have been approximately double the figures shown in Table 2.)

Table 3 Selected characteristics of women delivering in hospitals in the three strata

	High	Medium	Low
No.	3921	3988	3615
Registration status			
% not booked	44·6	26·6	11·9
% emergency admissions	17·9	6·1	10·4
Education			
Mean no. years completed	5·2	7·5	8·2
% with no education	27·7	17·8	7·2
% with more than 12 y.	3·2	9·9	14·0
Age at this delivery			
Mean age (±SD)	26·6±6·5	25·9±6·1	26·8±5·5
% less than 20	14·7	16·9	10·0
% 35 and over	14·4	9·7	8·6
No. of previous live births			
Mean parity (±SD)	2·2±2·8	1·5±2·2	1·2±1·8
% nulliparae	39·4	44·0	48·7
% with 4 or more	26·2	15·3	8·5
Antenatal care			
Mean no. of visits (± SD)	1·5±2·5	5·0±3·0	4·9±2·8
% with none	65·1	17·6	12·1
% with 7 or more	8·9	42·6	36·3
Other			
% with previous stillbirth	7·9	3·9	3·0
Mean interval since last			
pregnancy ended (months)	28·7	34·6	33·1
% with interval < 18 months	35·3	25·9	32·8

Table 3 shows that there were important differences among the patients in the three groups of hospitals. Patients in the high mortality hospitals were less likely to have received antenatal care and were more likely to be emergency admissions. They were also less well educated, more likely to be under 20 or over 35 years, were of higher parity, and were more likely to have had a previous stillbirth. In other words, the patients admitted to the hospitals with high mortality could be classified as being at high risk for a variety of reasons in addition to their breech presentations.

Table 4 shows that in terms of the obstetric characteristics, the patients in the high mortality hospitals were again more likely to be classified as being at high risk. They were much more likely to be anemic. They were more likely to exhibit delivery complications in

Table 4 Obstetric characteristics of patients in the three strata

	High	Medium	Low
Mean ($\pm$SD) Hb/100 ml	9·8±1·4	10·9±1·3	11·3±1·0
% Hb<10g/100 ml	30·4	14·9	4·5
% Hb not measured	37·8	50·0	40·8
% with *any* reported pathological antenatal condition	27·5	31·3	28·8
% with *any* additional complication	28·2	22·4	23·2
% with cord prolapse	2·9	1·5	1·5
% less than 36 weeks estimated gestation	15·0	13·5	8·4

Table 5 Selected obstetric management characteristics of hospitals in the three strata

	High	Medium	Low
No.	3921	3988	3615
Type of delivery			
Spontaneous	38·2	33·6	21·0
Breech extraction	38·0	28·7	30·0
Cesarean section	21·8	34·0	45·8
Other	2·1	3·8	3·3
Attendant at delivery			
Ob/Gyn physician	82·0	65·3	87·4
General physician	5·2	4·8	7·1
Medical student	5·3	11·8	1·0
Qualified midwife	4·9	15·6	3·1
Other	2·7	2·4	1·5
Anesthesia			
None	46·4	26·6	13·2
Local	18·2	29·3	13·5
Spinal or epidural	8·7	21·0	30·9
General	18·7	20·0	25·7
Other	7·9	3·1	16·7
Oxytocics			
None	91·9	80·9	88·8
Used for induction	0·7	1·4	2·7
Used for augmentation	7·4	17·7	8·5

addition to the breech presentation, and this includes a higher percentage of cord prolapse, a not infrequent complication of breech deliveries. Table 4 also shows that there were more short gestation babies in the high mortality group; however, it is often difficult to estimate gestational age and this is especially true in developing countries and in situations characterized by minimal antenatal care.

Another difference among the three groups requires comment. Table 4 shows that the highest mortality category has the lowest percentage of patients for which a pathological antenatal condition is reported. When it is recalled that almost two thirds of these patients had no antenatal care, it is not surprising that their antenatal conditions went unnoticed.

Table 5 shows that there were also important differences in the management of these deliveries among the three categories of hospitals. Patients delivering in the low mortality hospitals were about twice as likely to be delivered by cesarean as were patients delivering in the high mortality hospitals. Other management differences are largely associated with the difference in delivery technique, i.e. a greater use of general or spinal anesthesia, and a greater preponderance of physican-attended deliveries because of the greater preponderance of cesareans in the low mortality hospitals.

The mortality for all the breeches, regardless of the hospital group in which they were delivered, the method of delivery, their birth weight and the type of breech presentation was $78 \cdot 7$ per 1000 deliveries. The rate for the vaginally delivered babies was $103 \cdot 1$ compared with $30 \cdot 3$ for the abdominally delivered babies.

TYPE OF BREECH PRESENTATION

Table 6 shows the mortality for the babies according to whether they were delivered abdominally or vaginally, and the percentage delivered by cesarean section for the three different groups of hospitals, and according to the type of breech. In this and the following table, the relative risks shown are statistically significant ($p < 0 \cdot 05$), except where noted.

Footling breeches were the least likely to be delivered by cesarean in all three groups of hospitals; they also had the highest mortality. In the high mortality hospitals only $15 \cdot 2\%$ of the footling breeches were delivered abdominally, and their mortality was $47 \cdot 9$ per 1000 deliveries compared with 198·8 for the footlings delivered vaginally. At the other extreme, frank breeches were the most likely to be delivered by cesarean, almost one quarter (24·6%) in the high mortality hospitals, more than a third (34·9%) in the medium hospitals, and half (50·5%) in the low mortality hospitals. However, only in the low mortality hospitals was the mortality of the frank breeches lower than among the complete breeches. For the frank breeches delivered abdominally in the low mortality hospitals, the

Table 6 Percentage of breech babies delivered by cesarean section (CS), the mortality (per 1000 deliveries) of abdominally and vaginally delivered babies and the relative risk of vaginally delivered babies, by mortality level of the hospital where delivered, and by type of breech

Type of breech	Mortality level of hospital where delivered		
	High	Medium	Low
Frank Breech n=	1792	2160	2105
% delivered by CS	24·6	34·9	50·5
Mortality of CS deliveries	72·7	25·2	13·2
Mortality of vaginal deliveries	127·2	88·2	47·0
Relative risk	1·7	3·5	3·6
Mean gestation (SD)	38·1 (3·3)	37·9 (3·4)	38·7 (2·7)
Complete Breech n=	1168	931	829
% delivered by CS	23·1	36·4	44·0
Mortality of CS deliveries	51·8	38·4	13·7
Mortality of vaginal deliveries	115·8	77·7	71·1
Relative risk	2·2	2·0	5·2
Mean gestation (SD)	38·2 (3·2)	38·2 (3·4)	38·7 (2·9)
Footling Breech n=	961	897	681
% delivered by CS	15·2	29·7	32·2
Mortality of CS deliveries	47·9	30·1	22·8
Mortality of vaginal deliveries	198·8	101·4	77·9
Relative risk	4·2	3·4	3·4
Mean gestation (SD)	37·5 (3·8)	37·6 (3·5)	38·2 (3·2)
All Breech n=	3921	3988	3615
% delivered by CS	21·8	34·1	45·6
Mortality of CS deliveries	61·9	29·4	14·6
Mortality of vaginal deliveries	142·9	89·0	60·0
Relative risk	2·3	3·0	4·1
Mean gestation (SD)	38·0 (3·4)	37·9 (3·4)	38·6 (2·8)

mortality was only 13·2 per 1000 deliveries, compared with 47·0 per 1000 vaginally delivered frank breeches.

Whatever the overall level of mortality and for all types of breech presentation, those babies delivered by cesarean section had markedly improved survival. This relationship was most pronounced among the low mortality hospitals where the vaginally delivered babies had a level of mortality that was four times higher than the abdominally delivered babies, and least pronounced among the high mortality hospitals where the mortality of the vaginally delivered babies was twice as high as that of the abdominally delivered ones. In the hospitals with a medium level of overall mortality, the mortality of vaginally delivered breeches was three times that of those delivered by cesarean.

BIRTH WEIGHT

Table 7 shows a similar analysis but focuses on the weight of the breech neonates rather than the type of breech presentation. As expected, the percentage of very small (<1500 g) babies that was delivered by cesarean is small, only 5·0% and 10·9%, respectively, in the high and medium mortality hospitals, and even in the low mortality hospitals it is only 20·6%. The great majority of these babies died regardless of the method of delivery, and abdominal delivery provided no clear benefit. The mean estimated gestation of the babies weighing less than 1500 g was about 29 completed weeks in the three groups of hospitals.

Among the small babies (1500–2499 g), the percentage delivered abdominally increased to 14·5%, 28·7% and 33·2% in the three groups of hospitals. Abdominal delivery appeared to provide no benefit among the babies in the high mortality hospitals and only slight benefit in the medium mortality hospitals; only in the low mortality hospitals was the mortality of the vaginally delivered breeches as much as twice as high as that of the abdominally delivered babies.

The babies weighing 2500–3499 g constitute a majority (58·3%) of all the breech deliveries. The proportion delivered abdominally ranges from nearly a quarter (23·3%) in the high mortality hospitals to almost half (45·9%) in the low mortality hospitals, and in this weight group cesarean delivery appears to make more difference. In the high mortality hospitals the vaginally delivered babies had a level of mortality (81·5 per 1000) that is two and a quarter times that of the abdominally delivered infants (36·8 per 1000). The relationship is very

Table 7 Percentage of breech babies delivered by cesarean section (CS), the mortality (per 1000 deliveries) of abdominally and vaginally delivered babies and the relative risk of vaginally delivered babies, by mortality level of the hospital where delivered, and by birth weight

Birth weight	Mortality level of hospital where delivered		
	High	Medium	Low
< 1500 g n=	221	229	102
% delivered by CS	5·0	10·9	20·6
Mortality of CS deliveries	818·2	560·0	523·8
Mortality of vaginal deliveries	652·4	573·5	691·4
Relative risk	0·8*	1·0*	1·3*
Mean gestation (SD)	29·0 (3·4)	28·8 (3·8)	29·2 (4·5)
1500–2499 g n=	766	2703	419
% delivered by CS	14·5	28·7	33·2
Mortality of CS deliveries	171·2	69·3	43·2
Mortality of vaginal deliveries	178·6	117·8	92·9
Relative risk	1·0*	1·7	2·2
Mean gestation (SD)	35·6 (3·4)	35·9 (3·2)	36·2 (3·3)
2500–3499 g n=	2210	2312	2194
% delivered by CS	23·3	34·6	45·9
Mortality of CS deliveries	36·8	10·0	4·0
Mortality of vaginal deliveries	81·5	23·1	13·5
Relative risk	2·2	2·3	3·4
Mean gestation (SD)	39·1 (1·6)	39·1 (1·7)	39·1 (1·6)
> 3500 g n=	709	694	848
% delivered by CS	30·3	48·0	55·2
Mortality of CS deliveries	27·9	12·0	2·1
Mortality of vaginal deliveries	81·0	24·9	18·4
Relative risk	2·9	2·1	8·8
Mean gestation (SD)	39·7 (1·4)	39·6 (1·7)	39·8 (1·3)
Unknown birth weight n=	15	50	52
% delivered by CS	20·0	0·0	25·0
Mortality of CS deliveries	0·0	0·0	153·8
Mortality of vaginal deliveries	500·0	280·0	333·3
Relative risk	—	—	2·2*
Mean gestation (SD)	37·3 (3·6)	36·3 (5·4)	34·3 (5·4)

* Not statistically significant, $p >$ 0·05

similar in the medium mortality hospitals although the levels of mortality are lower (23·1 and 10·0 per 1000 deliveries). The difference is most pronounced in the low mortality hospitals where the mortality for both delivery types was very low – 13·5 per 1000 vaginally delivered babies and 4·0 per 1000 abdominally delivered babies.

Large babies (≥3500 g) often present the obstetrician with as many problems as very small babies, but this is perhaps less so for breech than vertex babies since head entrapment is less likely to occur with a large than with a small baby. Even in the high mortality hospitals almost one third (30·3%) of these babies were delivered by cesarean, and in the other two groups of hospitals the figures were 48·0% and 55·2%. In the high mortality hospitals there were 81·0 deaths per 1000 vaginally delivered babies compared with 27·9 deaths per 1000 abdominally delivered infants, a rate that was 2·9 times higher. In the medium mortality hospitals the respective rates were 24·9 per 1000 and 12·0 per 1000, the rate for the vaginal deliveries was twice that of the abdominal deliveries. In the low mortality hospitals, although the mortality of the vaginally delivered babies was almost nine times that of abdominally delivered babies, the mortality for both groups remained low (18.4 and 2·1, respectively).

For 117 cases (1%), the birth weight is unknown. The mean estimated gestation of these infants is similar to that of the infants weighing 2500–3499 g. The data for these babies are shown in Table 7, but no conclusions are drawn for this group.

Birth weight and type of breech presentation

When the different types of breech presentation are examined by birth weight, the frank and complete breeches tend to follow the same pattern we have already described. This is not the case, however, with the footlings. As expected, the footling breeches are slightly smaller than the frank or complete breeches, although the difference is not pronounced (26·3% weighed less than 2500 g compared with 19·7% of the frank and 19·9% of the complete breeches). The footling babies show benefit from cesarean delivery in both the small and the very small weight groups; however, two points should be remembered: first, mortality remains high for these babies whether they are delivered vaginally or abdominally and ranges from 714·3 per 1000 very small babies delivered vaginally in high mortality hospitals to 60·0 per 1000 small babies delivered abdominally in medium mortality hospitals. Second, none of the relative risks is statistically significant.

Additional analysis of these data will continue to focus on the interaction between birth weight and type of breech presentation on the outcome for the fetus, and will also examine the effect of maternal age and parity on the outcome of breech presentations.

MATERNAL DEATHS

Twenty mothers died, 1 in the low mortality hospitals, 5 in the medium and 14 in the high. Maternal mortality rates (per 1000 deliveries) were higher among women with cesarean than vaginal deliveries in the high mortality hospitals (7·0 compared with 2·6) and the medium mortality hospitals (2·2 compared with 0·8). The single maternal death in the low mortality hospital occurred with a vaginal delivery, giving a rate of 0·5 per 1000 deliveries compared with 0 for abdominal deliveries. The maternal mortality rate in the United States in 1978 and 1979 was 0·1 per 1000 live births (not deliveries)[1,27], but this figure includes deaths from all pregnancy-related causes, including ectopic pregnancy and abortion. It is likely that less than half the US figure is comparable with the rates found in this study, which speaks clearly to the problems of obstetrics in the Third World. Detailed death reports are available on 12 of these 20 deaths. Three of the 12 patients were admitted to hospital in good condition; the first of these underwent cesarean delivery (she had placenta previa in addition to the breech presentation) and died of cardiac arrest while still in the operating room. The general anesthesia was administered by an auxiliary nurse. The second came from a remote village with an intrauterine fetal death, she delivered a macerated fetus and the cause of death was attributed to shock and coagulation problems. The third case involved a placenta abruptio and some pre-existing kidney problems; cause of death was attributed to nephritis.

Deaths of the nine patients admitted in poor condition were attributed to the following causes: acute hepatic/renal failure (with antepartum hemorrhage), infection following subtotal hysterectomy for uterine rupture, hypovolemic shock following cesarean section for placenta previa (grand multipara), pleural effusion and postpartum hemorrhage after vaginal delivery (previous osteosarcoma), acute renal failure following subtotal hysterectomy for uterine rupture, eclampsia, hypovolemic shock following cesarean delivery for placenta previa, cerebral hemorrhage following cesarean delivery (patient was eclamptic and diabetic), acute peritonitis of unknown origin (patient died on day 9 after exploratory laparotomy and cesarean).

All of the cesarean patients among these deaths had indications for abdominal delivery in addition to the breech presentation. All patients who died, including those admitted in relatively good condition, had multiple medical problems.

SUMMARY AND CONCLUSIONS

This analysis confirms the conclusions of earlier researchers that, except for very small babies (less than 1500 g), cesarean delivery improves the chances of survival of breech babies. Furthermore, although it is generally true that the most improvement is made where there is more room for improvement, in this case the greatest gains are made where overall mortality is already low and where vaginally delivered breeches are most likely to survive, i.e. the low mortality hospitals.

However, with respect to the type of breech presentation, it is the footling that appears to derive the most benefit from abdominal delivery. When all three categories of hospitals are taken together, the mortality of vaginally delivered footlings is 3·6 times higher than that of abdominally delivered footlings, whereas with frank and complete breeches, the relative risks are 2·9 and 3·1 respectively.

With respect to birth weight, the relative risk is highest for the weight group over 3500 g and lowest for the very small (less than 1500 g) infants, implying that cesarean delivery provides no apparent benefit for these very small babies.

What recommendations for the physician can be drawn from this? It would appear that to abdominally deliver an infant of less than 1500 g is rarely worth the increased risk to the mother. If the baby weighs 1500–2499 g, there is marked improvement in survival only in those hospitals where overall mortality is already low (these are probably hospitals with facilities to care for the high-risk neonate). Normal weight babies, on the other hand, stand to benefit most from cesarean delivery and this is recommended (except where there are special contraindications) in almost all hospitals. Obviously this places on the physician the onus of estimating birth weight, often with inadequate means for estimation. The physican should continue to be aware of, and take into consideration such factors as the mother's future reproductive plans, the probability that her next delivery will occur in hospital, and the number of living children she already has. The additional maternal risk of abdominal delivery must be taken into account.

References

1 Advance Report of Final Mortality Statistics (1979). *NCHS Monthly Vital Statistics Report*, **31**(6), 10 (Suppl.) September 30, 1982

2 Bowes, W. A., Taylor, E. S., O'Brien, M. and Bowes, C. (1979). Breech delivery: evaluation of the method of delivery on perinatal results and maternal morbidity. *Am. J. Obstet. Gynecol.*, **135**, 965

3 Brenner, W. E. (1978). Breech presentation. *Clin. Obstet. Gynecol.*, **21**, 511

4 Brenner, W. E., Bruce, R. D. and Hendricks, C. H. (1974). The characteristics and perils of breech presentations. *Am. J. Obstet. Gynecol.*, **118**, 700

5 Chez, R. A., Rovinsky, J. J., Weingold, A. B. and Andros, G. J. (1977). Management of Breech Presentation. (Symposium) *Contemp. Obstet. Gynecol.*, **10**, 118

6 Collea, J. B., Chein, C. and Quilligan, E. J. (1980). The randomized management of term breech presentation: a study of 208 cases. *Am. J. Obstet. Gynecol.*, **137**, 235

7 Cruikshank, D. P. and Pitkin, R. M. (1977). Delivery of the premature breech. *Obstet. Gynecol.*, **50**, 367

8 De Crespigny, L. J. C. and Pepperell, R. J. (1970). Perinatal mortality and morbidity in breech presentation. *Obstet. Gynecol.*, **53**, 141

9 Duenhoelter, J. H., Wells, C. E., Reisch, J. S., Santos-Ramos, R. and Jimenez, J. M. (1979). A paired controlled study of vaginal and abdominal delivery of the low birth weight breech fetus. *Obstet. Gynecol.*, **54**, 310

10 Evrard, J. R. and Gold, E. M. (1977). Cesarean section and maternal mortality in Rhode Island: incidence and risk factors, 1965–1975. *Obstet. Gynecol.*, **50**, 594

11 Galloway, W. H., Bartholomew, R. A., Colvin, E. D., Grimes, W. H., Fish, J. S. and Lester, W. M. (1967). Premature breech delivery. *Am. J. Obstet. Gynecol.*, **99**, 975

12 Goldenberg, R. L. and Nelson, K. G. (1977). Viability and the premature fetus in distress. *Am. J. Obstet. Gynecol.*, **127**, 240

13 Hall, J. H., Kohl, S., O'Brien, F. and Ginsberg, M. (1965). Breech presentation and perinatal mortality. *Am. J. Obstet. Gynecol.*, **91**, 665

14 Hibbard, L. T. (1976). Changing trends in cesarean section. *Am. J. Obstet. Gynecol.*, **125**, 798

15 Karp, L. E., Doney, J. R., McCarthy, T., Meis, P. J. and Hall, M. (1979). The premature breech: trial of labor or cesarean section? *Obstet. Gynecol.*, **53**, 88

16 Kauppila, O. (1975). The perinatal mortality in breech deliveries and observations on affecting factors. A retrospective study of 2,227 cases. *Acta Obstet. Gynecol. Scand.* (Suppl. 39)

17 Lewis, B. V. and Seneviratne, H. R. (1979). Vaginal breech delivery or cesarean section. *Am. J. Obstet. Gynecol.*, **134**, 615
18 Lopez-Escobar, G., Riano-Gamboa, G., Fortney, J. and Janowitz, B. (1979). Breech presentations in a sample of Colombian hospitals. *Int. J. Gynaecol. Obstet.*, **17**, 284
19 Lyons, E. R. and Papsin, F. R. (1978). Cesarean section in the management of breech presentation. *Am. J. Obstet. Gynecol.*, **130**, 558
20 Mann, L. I. and Galant, J. M. (1979). Modern management of the breech delivery. *Am. J. Obstet. Gynecol.*, **134**, 611
21 Neilson, D. R. (1970). Management of the large breech infant. *Am. J. Obstet. Gynecol.*, **107**, 345
22 Petitti, D., Olson, R. O. and Williams, R. L. (1979). Cesarean section in California – 1960 through 1975. *Am. J. Obstet. Gynecol.*, **133**, 391
23 Placek, P. J. (1976). Maternal and infant health factors associated with low birth weight: findings from the 1972 natality survey. In Reed, D. M. and Stanley, F. S. (eds.) *The Epidemiology of Prematurity* (Baltimore: Urban & Schwarzenberg)
24 Rosen, M. G. (1981). The National Institutes of Health Consensus Development Statement on Cesarean Childbirth: A Summary. *J. Reprod. Med.*, **26**, 103
25 Rovinsky, J. J., Miller, J. A. and Kaplan, S. (1973). Management of breech presentation at term. *Am. J. Obstet. Gynecol.*, **115**, 497
26 Rubin, G. L., Peterson, H. B., Rochat, R. W., McCarthy, B. J. and Terry, J. S. (1981). Maternal death after cesarean section in Georgia. *Am. J. Obstet. Gynecol.*, **139**, 681
27 Sachs, B. P., McCarthy, B. J., Rubin, G., Burton, A., Terry, J. S. and Tyler, C. W. The case for and against a cesarean delivery for breech infants and low birth weight vertex infants. In preparation
28 *World Health Statistics 1981*, WHO, Geneva, 1981

Section III:
BIRTH SPACING:
DETERMINANTS AND
CONSEQUENCES

7
Child survivorship and pregnancy spacing in Iran

B. JANOWITZ and D. J. NICHOLS

It has been argued that declines in infant and childhood mortality are necessary before populations adjust their fertility downward. It follows that family planning programs will be increasingly successful as mortality declines, because more women will want to control the number of births they have. In an environment in which infant and child death rates are high, couples may compensate by having extra births in anticipation that some children will die[1,3]. Such a strategy discourages the use of contraception. Couples who actually suffer child loss may replace lost children; such couples will have a higher fertility than those whose children survive. Couples experiencing child loss may delay using contraceptives until the lost child has been replaced. Reduction in mortality will lessen the impact of these motivations for having children and raise the demand for contraception[6]. The effect of child survival on pregnancy intervals has been assessed and is examined in this chapter.

The data used in this study consist of over 15 000 records of hospital deliveries to women who report one or more previous pregnancies at what has, until recent events in Iran, been known as the Queen Farah Maternity Hospital in Tehran. This hospital participated in FHI's Maternity Care Monitoring study between July, 1977 and July, 1978.

The retrospective data collected on the Maternity Record are, of necessity, as reported by each individual respondent. In addition, many of the important questions concerning behavior during the pregnancy interval leading to the current delivery have more complex answers than are provided for in the questionnaire. Four examples with respect to key variables in the present investigation should be mentioned at the outset. First, there is only a single question on the Maternity Record about breast-feeding that combines information on whether a child was ever breast-fed and the length of breast-feeding. In addition, the duration of breast-feeding is categorized in intervals – none, <3 months, <6 months, etc – so that checks on data quality by examining patterns of heaping cannot be made. Also, the duration of breast-feeding is reported without concomitant reference to the initiation of supplemental feeding. Particularly when lactation is examined in the context of prolonging the period of postpartum amenorrhea, the qualitative nature of breast-feeding may be as critical in the relationship as the quantitative length.

Second, women are asked to indicate the contraceptive method used (if any) during the interval solely in its dichotomous sense: use versus non-use. No information is collected on the length and intensity of use, the reason for method discontinuation, or the practice of more than one method of contraception since the last pregnancy outcome.

Third, the length (in months) of the previous pregnancy interval is reported directly on the questionnaire rather than calculated from a reported date of a previous outcome. As might be expected, such a procedure results in substantial heaping in intervals of multiples of 12 months. For example, the data show that of the sample respondents having a second outcome within 5 years of the first, 49% reported pregnancy outcomes of *exactly* 12, 24, 36, 48 or 60 months. To the extent that this represents more than simple rounding to the nearest year (and to the extent it was differentially practiced by different sub-groups of the study population), biases may exist in the data on pregnancy intervals.

Fourth, age at death of nonsurviving children is not reported. Thus, the interrelationships between the cessation of breast-feeding (or failure to initiate breast-feeding) and the death of a child cannot be thoroughly analyzed.

Notwithstanding the above limitations, the data collected at Queen Farah Hospital appear to be of relatively good quality. As shown in Table 1, the average age of the over 15000 respondents is 25·6 years, a mean that varies very little according to the outcome of the previous pregnancy and the use of breast-feeding during the interval. Mean parity (prior to the present delivery) among all women is 2·78; the mean number of surviving children is 2·40.

Table 1 Selected characteristics, according to outcome of the last pregnancy and breast-feeding during the last pregnancy interval

	Total	Live birth			No. live birth
		Breast-feeding	No breast-feeding		
			Surviving	Deceased	
Mean age	26	26	25	25	25
Mean age at marriage	16	16	16	16	16
% some education	27	27	24	21	33
% urban	93	93	94	94	95
Mean parity	2·8	2·8	2·8	3·0	2·1
Mean living children	2·4	2·5	2·5	1·5	1·8
Mean child loss	0·4	0·4	0·4	1·5	0·3
Mean stillbirths/ spontaneous abortions	0·3	0·2	0·2	0·2	1·4
Mean interval (months)	38	41	35	21	20
% contracepting during interval	48	52	50	18	23
% wanting no additional children	63	66	65	37	48
% planning postpartum contraception	91	92	92	75	85
Among women who want no additional children	100	100	100	99	99
Among women who want additional children	73	75	76	59	69
% with current outcome surving	97	98	98	94	95
Number of women	15 403	12 004	1511	868	1020

The average pregnancy interval for the entire study population is 38 months, a reasonable figure for a group of women of whom nearly one half (48%) practiced contraception during the interval. Use of contraception varies only slightly with breast-feeding status for women with surviving previous outcomes. Women whose previous pregnancy resulted in other than a surviving live birth are substantially less likely to have used contraception and have pregnancy intervals averaging 21 months.*

---

* One indication of the quality of the data is the average *birth* interval of 21 months to women who neither breast-fed nor used any form of contraception during the interval (calculated from the data presented in Table 3). This finding is in keeping with other empirical studies that have found birth intervals for such women to be about 20 months[5], and is considerably shorter than birth intervals of 24–37 months calculated by Jain and Bongaarts[2] based on World Fertility Survey data.

PREGNANCY INTERVALS

Table 2 presents data on the average length of the last pregnancy interval by previous pregnancy outcome and breast-feeding status during the last pregnancy interval. Among women not breast-feeding, those whose last pregnancy ended in a live birth and whose last child is still living have, by far, the longest intervals (35·2 months). They are followed (in decreasing interval order) by women whose last pregnancy ended in a nonsurviving live birth, women whose last pregnancy ended in a stillbirth, and women with spontaneous abortions. The average intervals for such women are 21·4, 20·7 and 19·8 months, respectively. Among women who did breast-feed during the interval, surviving live births are also associated with far longer intervals (41·4 months versus 28·0 months) than nonsurviving outcomes.

Table 2 Mean length (in months) of the last pregnancy interval by outcome of the previous pregnancy and breast-feeding during the interval

Previous outcome	Total		No breast-feeding		Breast-feeding	
Live birth: surviving	40·7	(13 208)	35·2	(1511)	41·4	(11 697)
Live birth: deceased	23·1	(1175)	21·4	(868)	28·0	(307)
Stillbirth	20·7	(158)	20·7	(158)	—	—
Spontaneous abortion	19·8	(862)	19·8	(862)	—	—
Total	38·0	(15 403)	27·1	(3399)	41·1	(12 004)

CONTRACEPTION

Table 3 examines pregnancy intervals by contraceptive use and breast-feeding practices during the last pregnancy interval. This division allows the separation of the biologic effects, including the shortening of the period of pregnancy and breast-feeding, both of which affect the period of postpartum amenorrhea, and the motivational factors that work through contraceptive practices and sexual activity. Among women who did not breast-feed, those who did not contracept have the shortest intervals within categories of pregnancy outcome: differences between contraceptors and non-contraceptors vary from 19 to 24 months. Among women who did not contracept during the interval, those whose last pregnancy ended in a spontaneous abortion have the

Table 3 Mean length (in months) of the last pregnancy interval, by outcome of the previous pregnancy, and breast-feeding and contraception during the interval

Previous outcome	Non-contraceptors		Contraceptors	
No breast-feeding				
Live birth: surviving	23·4	(757)	47·1	(754)
Live birth: deceased	17·8	(716)	38·1	(152)
Stillbirth	17·3	(131)	36·3	(27)
Spontaneous abortion	15·2	(660)	34·6	(202)
Total	18·9	(2264)	43·4	(1135)
Breast-feeding				
Live birth: surviving	29·0	(5615)	52·9	(6082)
Live birth: deceased	22·8	(213)	39·7	(94)
Stillbirth	—	—	—	—
Total	28·8	(5828)	51·7	(6176)

shortest intervals since they have the shortest periods of postpartum amenorrhea. Women whose last pregnancy was full term but whose child died or was stillborn have longer pregnancy intervals. For these groups, biologic influences are similar, since all women experienced full-term pregnancies with no lengthening of the period of postpartum amenorrhea resulting from breast-feeding. Women whose last pregnancy ended in a live birth with the child still alive at the current delivery have substantially longer intervals. As these women neither breast-fed nor used contraception, how can this difference be explained? It is possible that some of the women with surviving live births practiced postpartum abstinence and did not consider such behavior to be contraception. In addition, problems associated with child care may have reduced coital frequency below that of women who are not caring for babies. Coital frequency may also be higher among those experiencing an unfavorable pregnancy outcome; such women are more likely to be trying to have another child as soon as possible.

Among contracepting women who do not breast-feed, those whose last pregnancy ended in a surviving child have longer pregnancy intervals than women whose child died or was stillborn or whose pregnancy ended in a spontaneous abortion. Women whose last pregnancy ended in a currently surviving live birth probably practice contraception more consistently than do other women. Women whose last child was born alive but subsequently died may cease practicing contraception or practice it less regularly after the child's death. Unfortunately, the available data are not sufficient to investigate these hypotheses further.

Among breast-feeding women, pregnancy intervals are longer for contraceptors than for noncontraceptors, with differences similar to those found for non-breast-feeding women. This result is surprising since it might have been expected that the impact of contraception on the length of the interval would be greater for non-breast-feeders. (In the section below, we control for length of breast-feeding to determine if these results were affected by different breast-feeding practices between these contraceptors and non-contraceptors.) Controlling for contraceptive use, we find longer pregnancy intervals among women with a surviving outcome. Part of this difference may be explained by more prolonged breast-feeding among mothers with a surviving child. The greater difference among contraceptors than among non-contraceptors in length of the interval by survival status may also be caused by earlier cessation of contraceptive use among women with a child who does not survive.

BREAST-FEEDING

In general, women who breast-fed and breast-fed for extended periods had longer pregnancy intervals than women who did not breast-feed (Table 4). Among contraceptors and non-contraceptors, the length of the pregnancy interval is affected by the duration of breast-feeding with the effect larger among the non-contraceptors. Even among the contraceptors, however, the pregnancy interval increases with the length of breast-feeding. The longer pregnancy interval for the non-breast-feeders than for women who breast-feed less than 6 months is difficult to explain. It may be that the women who do not breast-feed intend to breast-feed their babies but that the sickness of the baby or of the mother interferes with breast-feeding. (The failure to find any difference in age, education or parity between mothers who breast-feed and those who do not breast-feed [Table 1] supports this hypothesis.) Such an illness may impair fecundity and/or decrease sexual activity, thereby lengthening pregnancy intervals. When the length of the period of breast-feeding increases beyond 20 months, we find the most substantial effect on the length of the interval. This result is difficult to interpret. Breast-feeding will delay ovulation, but the

Table 4 Mean length (in months) of the last pregnancy interval, by duration of breast-feeding, contraceptive use during the interval, and survival status of the previous pregnancy outcome

Duration of breast-feeding	Total		Non-contraceptors		Contraceptors	
Live birth: surviving						
0 months	35·2	(1511)	23·4	(757)	47·0	(754)
1–5 months	32·9	(2182)	20·6	(1132)	46·2	(1050)
6–11 months	33·0	(1743)	22·6	(997)	46·8	(746)
12–14 months	35·4	(1660)	26·3	(932)	47·0	(728)
15–20 months	39·4	(1631)	28·7	(810)	50·0	(821)
21+ months	51·8	(4481)	39·8	(1745)	59·5	(2736)
Total	40·7	(13 208)	28·4	(6373)	52·2	(6835)
Live birth: deceased						
0 months	21·4	(868)	17·8	(718)	38·6	(150)
1–5 months	23·6	(173)	20·0	(127)	33·5	(46)
6–11 months	30·1	(75)	25·2	(56)	44·3	(19)
12+ months	38·2	(59)	30·1	(30)	46·6	(29)
Total	23·1	(1175)	19·0	(931)	39·1	(244)

longer breast-feeding is practiced, the more likely it is for menstruation to return. By 12 months, most mothers will either have stopped breast-feeding altogether or introduced food supplements to the baby's diet. These supplements will increase the probability that the woman resumes ovulation; *additional breast-feeding in such a context should not add substantially to her protection against pregnancy*. Nevertheless, we have found that the greater increases in the length of the pregnancy interval occur only when breast-feeding is prolonged. It may be that causation also runs in the opposite direction; women may continue to breast-feed until breast-feeding is restricted by pregnancy.

Among women with a live-born child that does not survive, the duration of breast-feeding is seen to affect the length of the pregnancy interval. Some of these differences in intervals may be affected by changes in patterns of sexual activity or contraceptive use that occur as a result of the child's death. Without information on age at death, though there is undoubtedly a positive correlation between the duration of breast-feeding and the age at death, it is not possible to study this relationship further.

CONTRACEPTION AND BREAST-FEEDING

How does the average length of the pregnancy interval of contracepting women compare with that of breast-feeding women? Table 4 makes these comparisons. Women who breast-feed without contracepting have shorter pregnancy intervals than women who breast-feed and contracept regardless of survival status of the child. Even when women breast-feed for extended periods, pregnancy intervals are still of shorter duration than for contracepting women. For example, women with a surviving child who use no contraception and breast-feed for at least 21 months have an average pregnancy interval of 39·8 months, while women who use contraception and do not breast-feed have an average interval of 47·0 months. Breast-feeding, it would seem, delays pregnancy, but contraception is more effective in delaying it.

If women use contraception throughout the period that they breast-feed, then breast-feeding should not affect the length of the pregnancy interval. But women may delay the initiation of contraception or cease contraception altogether (presumably when they wish to become pregnant) but continue breast-feeding. When such is the case, breast-feeding practices will affect the length of the pregnancy interval. Since it is only known whether contraception was practiced during the interval and not for how long, it is not possible to examine this hypothesis. It does appear, however, that breast-feeding, when combined with contraception, does extend the length of the pregnancy interval.

BIOLOGIC VERSUS MOTIVATIONAL FACTORS

The effects of biologic and motivational factors on pregnancy intervals may be studied by expanding on an approach suggested by Knodel[4]. We do this by looking at differences in the length of the third pregnancy interval according to the outcomes of the two previous pregnancies and the use of contraception in the interval between the second and third pregnancy. Among women whose second pregnancy ended in a live birth of a child still living, any differences in the length of the third pregnancy interval must be attributed to motivation unless there are systematic differences in breast-feeding. In our sample, there are some differences in breast-feeding practices associated with both survival

Table 5 Mean length (in months) of the third pregnancy interval, by outcomes of the two previous pregnancies and contraceptive use during the interval. Restricted to women with exactly two previous pregnancies

Previous outcomes		Total		Non-contraceptors		Contraceptors	
1st: 2nd:	surviving surviving	42·1	(2445)	29·4	(1099)	52·5	(1346)
1st: 2nd:	not surviving surviving	33·0	(518)	26·3	(333)	45·2	(185)
1st: 2nd:	surviving stillbirth or infant death	21·6	(171)	18·3	(137)	35·1	(34)
1st: 2nd:	not surviving stillbirth or infant death	17·9	(86)	16·8	(81)	34·8	(5)
1st: 2nd:	surviving spontaneous abortion	17·3	(140)	14·9	(111)	26·3	(29)
1st: 2nd:	not surviving spontaneous abortion	16·1	(44)	14·6	(40)	31·5	(4)
Total		37·7	(3404)	26·2	(1801)	50·7	(1603)

status of the first child and contraceptive practices. When survival status of the first child is controlled for, women who do contracept breast-feed longer than women who do not contracept, and (controlling for contraceptive use) women who have two surviving children breast-feed for longer periods than do women with only one survivor.* As a consequence, the effect of both contraception and child survival in lengthening the pregnancy interval is overstated.

With these limitations in mind, Table 5 illustrates that outcomes of previous pregnancies are associated with the length of the third pregnancy interval. Women with two living children have average pregnancy intervals nine months longer than women with one surviving child whose first child died or whose first pregnancy terminated in a stillbirth or spontaneous abortion. This difference is related to variations in contraceptive use. Women who have two living

---

* These results would indicate that breast-feeding is not used as a substitute for contraception in protecting against pregnancy. See Jain[2], who found a negative association between the duration of breast-feeding and contraceptive use in five countries, a positive association in two and none in the eighth country.

children are more likely to have used contraception in the last pregnancy interval than women whose first pregnancy ended unsuccessfully. Even among interval contraceptors, women with two surviving children have longer pregnancy intervals than women with only the second-born child surviving. It may well be that the latter group uses contraception for a shorter period or uses it more sporadically. Among non-contraceptors also, women with two living children have longer pregnancy intervals than women whose first pregnancy outcome did not result in a surviving child. It may be that women with only one living child have a higher coital frequency because they are actively trying to have another child and/or that women with child-care responsibilities have a lower coital frequency because of household responsibilities.

The much shorter third pregnancy intervals among women with a nonsurviving *second* outcome are the result of a combination of motivational *and* biologic factors favoring short intervals. Differences in postpartum amenorrhea, breast-feeding and contraceptive use are all involved. Within outcome categories, contraceptors have substantially longer intervals than non-contraceptors. Within contraceptive use categories, spontaneous abortions are associated with slightly shorter intervals than are stillbirths and infant deaths. *All* intervals, however, are shorter than those for women with a second pregnancy outcome that resulted in a *surviving* child.

REGRESSION ANALYSIS

Although the results discussed above illustrate the degree of variation in the length of the third pregnancy interval associated with previous outcomes and contraceptive use during the interval, they do not explicitly consider the effects of other variables in the relationship. To assess the relative impact of previous outcomes, contraceptive use and breast-feeding in prolonging the pregnancy interval, we use multiple regression analysis using dummy variables for categorical data.

We include in the regression equation variables to measure not only outcomes of previous pregnancies, breast-feeding and contraceptive use, but, in addition, age and education. Breast-feeding categories are the same as in previous tabulations. Pregnancy outcome categories are the same as in Table 5, except that some combining of first outcome categories was necessary to compute regressions for subgroups.

Women with a surviving birth as a second outcome are still classified according to first outcome. Grouping is done according to second outcome rather than number of survivors because our focus is on the survival status of the penultimate pregnancy and the subsequent pregnancy interval. Contraception is categorized as modern (IUD/orals), traditional (mostly rhythm/withdrawal), and none. Education is dichotomized into some or none; it has been shown that few women have received any schooling, and early findings (not shown) indicated that further disaggregation does not add to the explanatory power of the regression equation. Age enters the equation as a continuous variable.

Pregnancy outcomes

The first column of Table 6 shows that, even controlling for contraceptive use and breast-feeding status, previous pregnancy outcomes affect the length of the pregnancy interval. Among women completing their third pregnancy, those for whom the first outcome only is not surviving have intervals averaging nearly 2 months less than the index group of women with two surviving children. Those whose second outcome was full term but not surviving (e.g. stillbirth or deceased) have intervals that are 7 months shorter,* and those whose second pregnancy resulted in a spontaneous abortion report intervals more than 10 months shorter than the index group.†

   Columns 2–5 present corresponding results according to contraceptive use and breast-feeding during the interval. Among women who practiced neither contraception nor breast-feeding since the previous pregnancy outcome, the shortest intervals are for women whose last pregnancy ended in a spontaneous abortion. Intervals are shorter for women whose last child died than for women whose last child survived. This confirms the finding presented in Table 3 and shows that even when controls are introduced for age and education, pregnancy intervals are still longer for women with a surviving child.‡

* 7·3 months shorter if the first outcome is surviving; 7·1 months shorter if the first outcome is not surviving.
† 11·1 months shorter if the first outcome is surviving; 7·7 months shorter if the first outcome is not surviving.
‡ The gross difference between the group with two surviving children and the group with a nonsurviving first child followed by a spontaneous abortion is 26 months (42·1−16·1), whereas the net difference is 7·7 months.

As argued earlier, this effect may be explained by women with a non-surviving child actively seeking pregnancy and/or child-care activities reducing sexual activity among women with a surviving child.

Among women who did breast-feed but did not contracept, the outcome of the previous pregnancy does not affect the length of the subsequent interval (column 3). Women whose last child died do not have substantially different pregnancy intervals from women whose last child survived. Perhaps women who breast-feed have children who die at older ages than the children of women who are not breast-fed. Thus, the impact of a child death on the pregnancy interval would vary by regression equation as the inclusion of women with children dying at different ages changed. As the age at death of nonsurviving children was not reported, this hypothesis cannot be tested.

The fourth column in Table 6 presents results for women who used contraception but did not breast-feed since the previous pregnancy. Differences in the length of the interval among outcome groups are quite large. It is very probable that contraceptive use varies greatly by women according to pregnancy outcome, but that the dichotomous contraceptive use variable used herein does not adequately capture this difference. Thus, reported differences are greater in column 4 than in column 2. Women with surviving pregnancy outcomes probably practice contraception more consistently and effectively than do women with nonsurviving outcomes, and many women whose child died probably cease contracepting to become pregnant once again.

Column 5 in Table 6 shows that, among women who contracepted *and* breast-fed, women whose last pregnancy ended in a child death have pregnancy intervals 9–11 months shorter than women whose last child survived. These results are similar to those found in column 4, again indicating that contraceptive use may have a greater impact on the length of the pregnancy interval than can be adequately measured with our available data.

Contraception

For other variables, the results show that contraceptive use has a large effect on the length of the pregnancy interval. For all women (column 1), modern contraceptors have pregnancy intervals 20 months longer than women who did not contracept, and users of traditional methods have intervals 17 months longer than women who did not contracept.

Table 6 Effects of previous pregnancy outcomes, contraceptive use, breast-feeding and other variables on the length of the third pregnancy interval for selected groups of women with exactly two previous pregnancies

Variable	All women	Breast-feeding and contraception during the interval			
		Neither .	B only	C only	Both
	(1)	(2)	(3)	(4)	(5)
Previous outcomes					
1st: surviving					
2nd: surviving	exc	exc	exc	exc	exc
1st: not surviving					
2nd: surviving	−1·6*	−4·4	0·4	−4·3	−2·5
1st: all outcomes					
2nd: stillbirth: deceased	−7·3*	−7·2*	−3·6	−12·4*	−11·4*
1st: all outcomes					
2nd: spontaneous abortion	−10·3*	-9·2*	a	−19·2*	a
Breast-feeding					
None	exc	a	a	a	a
1–5 months	0·2	a	exc	a	exc
6–11 months	0·3	a	2·2*	a	−2·1
12–14 months	2·0	a	5·0*	a	−1·1
15–20 months	4·3*	a	8·2*	a	−0·3
21+months	10·6*	a	15·0*	a	6·1*
Contraception					
None	exc	a	a	a	a
Traditional	16·8*	a	a	exc	exc
Modern	20·4*	a	a	3·6	4·3*
Education					
None	exc	exc	exc	exc	exc
1+years	1·2	−1·3	−0·6	1·1	3·8*
Age	1·6*	0·5*	1·0*	2·5	2·5*
R^2	0·47	0·18	0·28	0·27	0·21
n	3404	506	1295	213	1390

exc=excluded category for each set of dummy variables in the regression equation
a=inapplicable
* significant at 0·05 level

Results from Table 5 show that the difference in pregnancy interval between contraceptors and non-contraceptors is 24·5 months (50·7−26·2). Adjusting for the effects of survival status, education, etc, therefore, reduced this difference, as these variables explain why contraceptive use varies, but does not eliminate the difference.

Breast-feeding

What effect does breast-feeding have on lengthening the pregnancy interval? Women in Tehran who breast-fed for longer periods (21 months or more) have pregnancy intervals almost a year longer than women who breast-fed for less than 6 months; women who breast-fed for moderate periods (12–20 months) have pregnancy intervals only 2–4 months longer than women who did not breast-feed.

As in other studies in which duration of breast-feeding enters the regression as an independent variable, the direction of causation is not clear. A pregnancy interval cannot be shorter in length than the period of breast-feeding so that longer pregnancy intervals may facilitate for breast-feeding.

One way of adjusting for this effect is to compare the increase in the length of the pregnancy interval associated with an increase in breast-feeding by contraceptive use status. Among women who contracept, breast-feeding does not affect the length of the pregnancy interval until it is carried out for at least 21 months. Since virtually all women should have added supplementary food by this time this is precisely the period in which the 'protective' effect of breast-feeding should be reduced.

Turning to the non-contracepting women, we may conclude that effects are real through the 15–20 month group, but are probably over-estimated by about 6 months (the coefficient for the contracepting group) for the breast-feeding duration group 21 + months, implying that the time coefficient is 8·9 months rather than 15·0, which would suggest that the additional protection after breast-feeding for 15–20 months is less than a full month.

Among women who do not contracept, breast-feeding has a quantitatively greater effect on pregnancy intervals than among women who contracept. For women who contracept, breast-feeding can only increase the pregnancy interval if contraception is practiced inefficiently or use is terminated early. Therefore, it would be expected that the impact of breast-feeding would have a greater effect on pregnancy intervals for women who did not contracept compared with women who contracepted. Thus, it is not surprising to find that only very prolonged breast-feeding (21 + months) has an impact on the length of the pregnancy interval among contraceptors. If additional data on contraceptive use were available, including information on length of use, then differences in the impact of breast-feeding on the length of the pregnancy interval might be expected to vary even more by contraceptive status.

Pregnancy intervals are affected by contraceptive use, breast-feeding practices and pregnancy outcome. These three factors do not, however, act independently of one another but jointly in a relatively complex manner. If a child is not born alive or dies soon after birth, breast-feeding is not practiced or ceases. Women whose penultimate child survived are more likely to have contracepted in the previous pregnancy interval than are women without a survivor. Even when these two factors are adjusted for, pregnancy outcome still influences the length of the subsequent pregnancy interval.

These results may be useful in evaluating the impact of public health programs striving to reduce infant and childhood mortality. These programs will be more effective in increasing the interval between pregnancies (1) the greater the impact a rise in child survival has on increasing the rate of contraceptive use, and (2) the more widespread is breast-feeding, and particularly prolonged breast-feeding.

References

1 Chowdhury, A., Khan, A. and Chen, L. (1978). Experience in Pakistan and Bangladesh. In Preston, S. H. (ed.). *The Effects of Infant and Child Mortality on Fertility*, (New York: Academic Press)
2 Jain, A. R. and Bongaarts, J. (1981). Breastfeeding: patterns, correlates and fertility effects. *Stud. Fam. Plann.*, **12**, 79
3 Knodel, J. (1977). Breast-feeding and population growth. *Science*, **198**, 1111
4 Knodel, J. (1978). European populations in the past: family-level relations. In Preston, S. H. (ed.). *The Effects of Infant and Child Mortality on Fertility*, (New York: Academic Press)
5 Leridon, H. (1977). *Human Fertility: The Basic Components*. (Chicago: University of Chicago Press)
6 Omran, A. R. (1971). Health benefits of family planning. Presented at the *World Health Organization Scientific Group on Human Development and Public Health Meeting*, Geneva

8
Infant and child survival and contraceptive use in the closed pregnancy interval

B. JANOWITZ and D. J. NICHOLS

This chapter examines the link between the survival status of previous children and the decision to contracept. Women who have lost a child or children may be expected to have greater motivation to have another child, and hence be less likely to practice contraception than women whose children are all surviving. More recent losses may be associated with lower levels of interval contraception, as they are less likely to have been 'replaced' by a subsequent birth.

While other studies have examined the relationship between child survival and contraceptive use, they do not consider the impact of the sequence of child mortality on the practice of family planning[1,3,6,7-9]. Although summary data on the number of non-surviving offspring may be useful in studies in which mortality is a *dependent* variable, it is less relevant when used to predict or classify cases according to reported subsequent behavior.

A principal reason for this neglect may be the unavailability of the comparatively large data sets required to permit the disaggregation of a respondent's reported child loss into birth order categories, as well as the total number. Furthermore, contraceptive use among older women is less likely to be affected by the survival status of previous pregnancy outcomes than it is for younger women, as the former have had greater opportunity to adjust their fertility to these past outcomes. The present study fills a gap in the literature on childhood mortality and family planning by considering how the birth order of non-surviving outcomes affects contraceptive use.

SOURCE OF DATA

The data used in this chapter, as in the preceding one, consist of records of hospital deliveries to women at what has been known as the Queen Farah Maternity Hospital in Tehran. During the period between July 1977 and July 1978, data for over 20 000 deliveries are available from the Tehran hospital with over 15 000 women reporting at least one previous pregnancy. This analysis is restricted to the 10 245 cases in which women report one, two or three previous pregnancies. For each of the women, information on past pregnancy outcomes, contraceptive use and breast-feeding practices in the closed interval and current plans for additional children and contraceptive intentions are available.

First, women are asked to indicate the contraceptive method (if any) used during the interval. No information is collected on the length or frequency of use, contraceptive status at the onset of the pregnancy, the switching of methods or use of more than one method since the last pregnancy outcome. Age at death for non-surviving children is not reported. Therefore, it is not possible to document if the death of a child results in the cessation of contraception. In addition, women who planned no additional pregnancies and successfully contracepted are excluded altogether, since the data set includes only women with closed intervals. Thus, the results cannot be generalized to all women in the fertile ages.

BACKGROUND CHARACTERISTICS ACCORDING TO THE NUMBER OF PREVIOUS PREGNANCIES

Table 1 presents information on the background characteristics of women with one, two or three previous pregnancies delivering at the hospital. Women who have had more pregnancies are older and less educated than women with fewer pregnancies. The percentage of women whose last pregnancy ended in a stillbirth or spontaneous abortion or whose child subsequently died (non-surviving outcomes) does not vary with gravidity.* The percentage of women with one or more non-surviving outcomes is twice as great for women with two, and three times as great for women with three, than for women with one previous pregnancy. This result also indicates that survival is independent of the number of previous pregnancies. The mean number of surviving children rises with the number of pregnancies (the average number of sons is about half the average number of living children), and the average number of non-survivors is 0·14, 0·16 and 0·17 per pregnancy for women with one, two and three previous pregnancies. The data thus show no relationship between number of pregnancies and pregnancy loss.

Table 1   Selected characteristics according to the number of previous pregnancies (Women delivering at Queen Farah Hospital, Tehran, Iran: July 1977–July 1978)

	Previous pregnancies		
	1	*2*	*3*
Number of women	4284	3426	2535
Mean age (years)	21·0	23·4	26·1
% with some education	40·8	31·3	25·1
% urban	93·0	92·8	91·4
% previous outcome not surviving	14·3	13·3	12·7
% 1 or more nonsurviving outcomes	14·3	28·3	39·4
Mean number surviving children	0·86	1·68	2·50
Mean number surviving sons	0·45	0·85	1·25

CONTRACEPTIVE USE IN THE PREGNANCY INTERVAL

In Table 2 we present data on contraceptive use in the last pregnancy interval according to selected variables. In general, the survivorship of previous outcomes is found to be more highly related to contraceptive use than are such socio–demographic background variables as age, education and residence.† Within groups according to the number of

* Because of the presumed differences in motivation in the interval following an induced abortion, the few women (19 cases, or less than one fifth of one per cent) reporting such a penultimate outcome have been excluded from the analysis.
† A chi-square statistic was used to test separately for differences in contraceptive use according to categories of previous pregnancy outcome, surviving children, surviving sons, infant deaths, age, education and residence. Additionally, a test for a linear trend in proportions contracepting was used for surviving children, surviving sons and infant deaths. The 0·01 level of significance is used throughout.

Table 2 Reported rate of contraceptive use during the closed interval according to the number of previous pregnancies and selected variables (Women delivering at Queen Farah Hospital, Tehran, Iran: July 1977–July 1978)

	Previous pregnancies					
	1		2		3	
Total	·36	(4284)	·47	(3426)	·54	(2535)
Previous outcome						
Live, surviving	·42	(3671)	·52	(2968)	·58	(2218)
Live, not surviving	·07	(354)	·17	(244)	·26	(179)
Stillbirth	·05	(69)	·08	(25)	·39	(18)
Spontaneous abortion	·03	(190)	·18	(189)	·31	(120)
Surviving children						
0	·06	(613)	·08	(136)	·06	(33)
1	·42	(3671)	·30	(833)	·32	(203)
2	—		·55	(2457)	·48	(763)
3	—		—		·62	(1536)
Surviving sons						
0	·30	(2381)	·37	(1153)	·38	(509)
1	·44	(1903)	·50	(1642)	·54	(1081)
2	—		·58	(631)	·64	(755)
3	—		—		·64	(190)
Infant deaths						
0	·39	(3944)	·51	(2901)	·59	(1920)
1	·07	(340)	·27	(465)	·44	(507)
2	—		·03	(60)	·22	(98)
3	—		—		·00	(10)
Education						
None	·28	(2535)	·42	(2353)	·51	(1899)
1–4 years	·41	(267)	·60	(235)	·67	(159)
5–6 years	·51	(1033)	·61	(663)	·63	(400)
7 or more years	·47	(449)	·49	(175)	·66	(77)
Age						
Less than 25	·35	(3746)	·43	(2234)	·43	(937)
25–34	·46	(517)	·55	(1137)	·61	(1466)
35–45	·43	(21)	·46	(55)	·62	(132)
Residence						
Urban	·37	(3986)	·48	(3178)	·55	(2316)
Rural	·27	(298)	·42	(248)	·53	(219)

Number of cases in parentheses

previous pregnancies, women whose last birth is currently surviving are significantly more likely to have used contraception during the closed interval than women with non-surviving outcomes (child death, stillbirth or spontaneous abortion). Differences in contraceptive use among the non-surviving categories, however, are not significant.

Independent of the number of previous pregnancies, contraceptive use is significantly associated with the overall number of surviving children, the number of surviving sons and the number of infant deaths. Use increases with surviving children and surviving sons, and decreases with infant deaths. Figures 1–3 graphically depict these relationships. We used a test for a linear trend in proportions to confirm the statistical significance of all linear associations.

Education is also found to have a measurable effect on contraceptive use. Women with no education are significantly less likely to have practiced contraception during the interval than are women with one or more years of schooling. Among women with some education, however, additional years of schooling are associated with varying patterns of contraceptive use; this finding is observed in all three previous pregnancy categories. Age also has a significant impact on contraceptive use, although as with education the pattern of association varies according to the number of previous pregnancies.

Finally, urban women are somewhat more likely to have contracepted than rural women, although the difference is found to be significant only for those with one previous pregnancy.

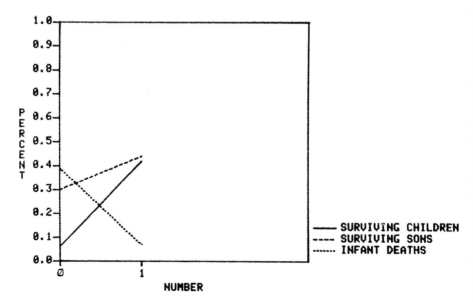

Figure 1   Contraceptive use: one previous pregnancy

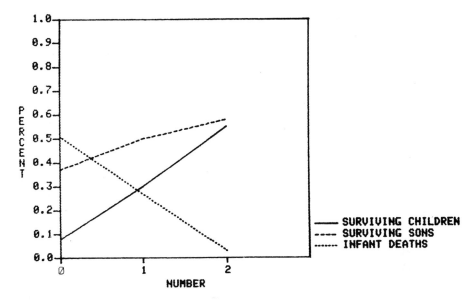

Figure 2   Contraceptive use: two previous pregnancies.

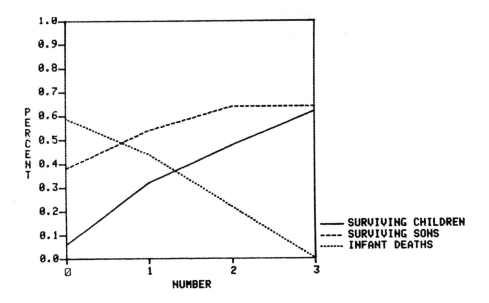

Figure 3   Contraceptive use: three previous pregnancies

Adjusted probabilities of contraceptive use

To examine the effects of pregnancy outcome, education, age and other variables in affecting the probability that a woman contracepted in the closed interval, we use multiple regression analysis. Pregnancy outcomes are divided into groups based on the number and order of surviving children. Non-surviving outcomes may be stillbirths or spontaneous abortions or live-born infants not surviving to the most recent delivery. Order of survival is distinguished according to whether the last pregnancy (prior to that leading to the current outcome) ended in a death and the number of non-surviving *previous* outcomes. Outcomes for all but the last pregnancy are therefore divided into categories based on the number surviving but not the order of survival.

CHILD SURVIVAL

Differences in the outcome of previous pregnancies have a significant effect on the probability that a woman contracepted during the last pregnancy interval. Considering first women who have had exactly one previous pregnancy (Table 3), we find that women with a surviving child have a probability 31 percentage points above that of women without a surviving child of having contracepted during the interval between pregnancies. The adjusted rate* of contraceptive use (Table 4) is 0·09 (or 9%) if the woman does not have a surviving child and 0·40 if she has a surviving child. For women with two previous pregnancies, the adjusted probability that a woman contracepted during the last pregnancy interval varies from a low of 0·17 for women with no surviving children to a high of 0·54 for women with two living children.

* The results of multiple regression may be described not only in terms of regression coefficients but also in terms of 'adjusted rates of contraceptive use.' There is an adjusted rate of contraceptive use corresponding to every dummy variable. Each adjusted rate is interpreted as an estimate of what contraceptive use would have been had these women been 'average' in terms of all other sets of dummy and continuous variables in the multiple regression. Thus, in the following example, the net regression coefficients for all sets of variables, except previous pregnancy outcome, are used to standardize the rate of contraceptive use. Adjusted rates of contraceptive use by pregnancy outcome for women who are average with respect to all other variables can be compared. The procedure used to calculate these rates is described by Bowen and Finegan[2].

Table 3 Regression coefficients of previous pregnancy outcomes and other variables on contraceptive use in the preceding pregnancy interval (Women delivering at Queen Farah Hospital, Tehran, Iran: July 1977–July 1978)

Surviving children	Previous pregnancies		
	1	2	3
Surviving children			
1: Last not surviving		·06	·05
1: Last surviving	·31*	·21*	·11
2: Last not surviving			·01
2: Last surviving		·37*	·21*
3			·25*
(reference category: 0 surviving)			
Proportion of pregnancies resulting in a surviving son	·04*	·08*	·20*
Age	·03*	·02*	·02*
Urban residence	·08*	·09*	·03
Education			
1–4 years	·16*	·20*	·18*
5–6 years	·23*	·22*	·17*
7+years	·18*	·12*	·21*
(reference category: 0 years)			
Constant	− ·62	− ·40	− ·26
R^2 (adjusted)	·14	·12	·10
Number of women	4284	3426	2535

* $p < 0.05$

Among women with three pregnancies, the adjusted probability of having contracepted during the last pregnancy interval varies from a low of 0·29 for women with one survivor (other than the last) to a high of 0·59 for women with three survivors. The adjusted rate for women with no surviving children (0·34) is found to be slightly higher than that for the former group, although the difference is not statistically significant.

Both the number of surviving children and the order of survival affect contraceptive use. Consider first the impact of number of survivors. Results for women with two or three previous pregnancies show that when the last child is still alive, the probability of having contracepted during the last interval increases with the number of surviving children. Adjusted rates of contraceptive use for women with two previous pregnancies are, respectively, 0·38 and 0·54 for

Table 4 Adjusted rate of contraceptive use during the closed interval according to the number and order of surviving children (Women delivering at Queen Farah Hospital, Tehran, Iran: July 1977–July 1978)

Surviving children	Previous pregnancies 1		2		3	
0	·09	(613)	·17	(136)	·34	(33)
1						
Last not surviving	—		·23	(322)	·29	(88)
Last surviving	·40	(3671)	·38	(511)	·45	(115)
2						
Last not surviving	—		—		·35	(196)
Last surviving	—		·54	(2457)	·55	(567)
3	—		—		·59	(1536)

Number of cases in parentheses

women with one and two surviving children. If the last child has died, reported differences are smaller: 0·17 and 0·23 for women with none versus one surviving child. Similarly, among women with three previous pregnancies, adjusted rates of contraceptive use are 0·45, 0·55 and 0·59 for women with one, two and three surviving children (including the last). If the last child has died, reported differences are smaller: 0·34, 0·29 and 0·35 for women with none, one and two surviving children.

The order of survival also influences past contraceptive behavior. Of women with two previous pregnancies but one surviving child, those whose second child is alive are much more likely to have contracepted than women whose first child is still alive (0·38 versus 0·23). Among women with three previous pregnancies, women whose last child is still alive are more likely to have contracepted than women whose last child has died (0·55 versus 0·35 for women with two surviving children and 0·45 versus 0·29 for women with one survivor). It is likely that considerations regarding the spacing of children account, at least in part, for these results. Women with one surviving child from two pregnancies (or those with two survivors from three pregnancies) may want the same number of additional children, no matter what the order of survival, but women whose second (or third) child died may wish to have that child sooner than women whose first (or second) child died.

SEX COMPOSITION

Not only does the number and order of surviving pregnancy outcomes affect contraceptive use, but also the number of sons is important in affecting contraceptive use. We measure sex composition as the percentage of women with some given number of living sons.* If women desire sons more than daughters, or at least wish to reach some target number of sons, then an increase in the proportion of women who have some given number of sons should result in an increase in the use of contraception.

Among women who have had exactly one pregnancy, the proportion with a living son is 0·45. This corresponds to a sex ratio of 0·52 (0·45 divided by 0·86) since only 86% of the women have a living child. If this child is a boy, then the mother's likelihood of having contracepted is 0·04 higher than that of a woman who did not have a surviving son (the probability of having contracepted would be 0·38 if she had a boy and 0·34 if she did not have a boy) (Table 5). Of women who have had two or three pregnancies, the probability of having contracepted during the last pregnancy interval also varies directly with the number of surviving sons. Clearly, the desire for sons is a

Table 5 Adjusted rate of contraceptive use during the closed interval according to the number of previous pregnancies and the number of surviving sons (Women delivering at Queen Farah Hospital, Tehran, Iran: July 1977–July 1978)

Surviving sons	Previous pregnancies		
	1	*2*	*3*
0	·34 (2381)	·44 (1153)	·45 (509)
1	·38 (1903)	·48 (1642)	·52 (1081)
2	—	·52 (631)	·59 (755)
3	—	—	·63 (190)

Number of cases in parentheses

* This measure is used in preference to a series of categorical variables that measure the number of sons or the sex distribution of a family because it is necessary to include a category 'no living sons.' Inclusion of this category is impossible since this is a category in the pregnancy outcome variable. If included here, linear dependence would result. The measure actually used suffers from the deficiency that the variable, sons, is not strictly continuous since children come in discrete units. Also, there may be non-linearities in the effect of changing numbers of male children on the use of contraception.

factor depressing contraceptive use. Consequently, women who have been 'successful' in having sons are more likely to have contracepted than women who have fewer or no sons.

OTHER VARIABLES

Women with some education are more likely to have contracepted than women with no education, but among women who have some education, there is no consistent relationship between the amount of schooling and contraceptive use.

Women residing in urban areas are more likely to have contracepted than rural women, but this variable is statistically significant only for women with one or two previous pregnancies.

Older women are more likely to have contracepted than younger women, and the effect of age is stronger for women with one previous pregnancy than for women with two or three. For women with one pregnancy, each additional year of age raises the probability that a woman contracepted by $0 \cdot 026$, so a difference in age of 10 years implies a difference in contraceptive use of $0 \cdot 26$. At higher gravidities, each additional year of age raises the probability of having contracepted by $0 \cdot 017$, so a difference in age of 10 years implies a difference of $0 \cdot 17$ in the probability of having contracepted.

APPLICABILITY OF THE MODEL

To determine how well the model fits the data, we have compared actual rates of contraception with adjusted rates.* In cases in which the actual rate of contraceptive use is above $0 \cdot 10$, the model fits the data extremely well (Table 6). These are also the cases in which women have at least one surviving child. Among women with no surviving children, the percentage of women contracepting is low and the model does not fit the data well.† The poorest fit is for the case of women with three pregnancies and no surviving children; the model predicts that 34% of the women are contraceptors when, in fact, only 6% actually

---

* To make these comparisons, we used the adjusted rates in Table 4 weighted by the percentage of women in the appropriate subgroups.
† This is to be expected and agrees with findings of other investigators[4,5] who suggest the use of a different regression model in instances in which the dependent variable is so highly skewed.

are. There are only 33 women in this group and the results, therefore, show that the 'fit' of the model is particularly poor when there is a very small number of cases combined with a very low percentage of women practicing contraception.

Table 6 Adjusted and actual rates of contraceptive use according to the number of previous pregnancies and surviving children (Women delivering at Queen Farah Hospital, Tehran, Iran: July 1977–July 1978)

Surviving children	Previous pregnancies		
	1	2	3
0	·09 (·06)	·17 (·08)	·34 (·06)
1	·40 (·42)	·32 (·30)	·38 (·32)
2	—	·54 (·55)	·50 (·48)
3	—	—	·59 (·62)

Actual rates in parentheses next to adjusted rates

IMPLICATIONS

The use of contraception in the closed pregnancy interval is dependent on the survival status of previous pregnancies, especially the penultimate pregnancy. Women who had more favorable pregnancy outcomes – surviving children – are more likely to have contracepted than women who have had at least one pregnancy (particularly the penultimate) end unfavorably.

To assess the impact of increased survivorship on contraceptive practice in the study population, we have calculated hypothetical prevalence rates based on 25% and 50% reductions in mortality of the last pregnancy outcome (Table 7). The procedure utilizes the adjusted group-specific rates presented in Table 4, but applies them to different distributions of survivors.* Even with such substantial – and, in the short run, unlikely – reductions in infant and child mortality, it may be

* The calculation assumes improved survivorship only at the *last* pregnancy outcome, and leaves unchanged the effect of child loss resulting from antecedent pregnancies. For example, among women with three previous pregnancies (Table 4), it may be seen that a total of 1732 women had two surviving children at the time of the third delivery: 196 for whom the third outcome was *not* surviving, and 1536 for whom it was. A 25% improvement in survivorship thus reduces the former group by 49, and adds that number to the latter. Adjusted rates from Table 4 are applied, and result in the proportions presented in Table 7.

Table 7   Adjusted rate of contraceptive use during the closed interval, assuming 25% and 50% reductions in mortality of the last pregnancy outcome (Women delivering at Queen Farah Hospital, Tehran, Iran: July 1977–July 1978)

	Previous pregnancies		
	1	2	3
Reported level*	·36	·47	·54
25% reduction	·37	·48	·55
50% reduction	·38	·49	·56

* From Table 2

seen that overall contraceptive prevalence increases only negligibly. We offer the following explanation for this apparent 'inelasticity' of contraceptive use. Since about 87% of the last pregnancy outcomes are already surviving, even as much as a 25% reduction in mortality will result in a corresponding increase in survivorship to only 90%. Thus, the higher rates of contraceptive use among women with surviving (versus non-surviving) last outcomes are not applied to a great number of individuals, thus changing the overall prevalence only slightly.

Notwithstanding the minor effect of improved survivorship on aggregate contraceptive use rates, the impact at the individual level is considerable. Women with a surviving last outcome are from one and one half to over four times as likely to have used family planning in the closed interval following the first, second or third birth as women with a non-surviving outcome. Particularly in societies with high rates of infant and child mortality, then, it follows that programs which improve child survivorship will effectively result in higher rates of contraception and lower fertility for that sub-group of women whose children may otherwise have died.

References

1 Aghajanian, A. and Mehryar, A. (1979). Effect of child mortality on contraceptive use in rural Iran. *Eugenics Soc. Bull.*, **11**, 14

2 Bowen, A. and Finegan, O. (1969). *The Economics of Labor Force Participation*, p. 641. (Princeton, NJ: Princeton University Press)

3 Hashimoto, J. and Hongladarom, C. (1981). Effect of child mortality on fertility in Thailand. *Economic Development and Cultural Change*, **29**, 781

4 Hermalin, A. *et al.* (1979). Do intentions predict fertility? The experience in Taiwan, 1967–74. *Stud. Fam. Plann.*, **10**, 75

5 Nerlove, M. and Press, S. (1973). *Univariate and Multivariate Log–Linear and Logistic Models.* (Santa Monica, CA: Rand Corporation)

6 Pebley, A., Delgado, H. and Brinemann, E. (1979). Fertility desires and child mortality experience among Guatemalan women. *Stud. Fam. Plann.*, **10**, 129

7 Rutstein, S. and Medica, V. (1979). The Latin American Experience. In Preston, S. (ed.). *The Effects of Infant and Child Mortality on Fertility*, (New York: Academic Press)

8 Scrimshaw, S. (1978). Infant mortality and behavior in the regulation of family size. *Pop. Devel. Rev.*, **4**, 383

9 Taylor, D., Newman, J. and Kelly, N. (1976). The child survival hypothesis. *Pop. Stud.*, **30**, 263

9

The effect of birth interval on perinatal survival and birth weight

J. A. FORTNEY and J. E. HIGGINS

It has long been recognized, at least in developing countries, that short birth intervals have a negative effect on the well-being of the mother and of the infant displaced by the new pregnancy. In some cultures this knowledge is internalized to the extent that it is incorporated into the language; 'kwashiokor', in one of the languages of Ghana, means a disease occurring in a young child displaced from his mother's breast by a new baby[15]. In many areas of Africa, the baby who displaced his older sibling is called a thief[14]. Because of this, many cultures have established practices that serve to delay a new pregnancy at least until the baby is weaned; prolonged breast-feeding is accompanied by sexual abstinence in many societies[10]. Sometimes abstinence is maintained until the resumption of menstruation or longer[2].

Less easily understood is the effect of the short birth interval on the new infant. While it is easy to understand the difficulties of a mother with two (or more) babies close together and to hypothesize the consequences of some of those difficulties[8,11] (such as increased infant and child mortality), it is less obvious why infants should show an immediate effect of short birth interval as evidenced by higher perinatal mortality, higher fetal wastage and lower birth weight. Nevertheless, several studies have shown this to be the case. Nearly 40 years ago, Eastman[4] studied 5158 second or later children born at the Johns Hopkins University Hospital, Baltimore, MD, between 1936 and 1943 and found that babies born after a short pregnancy interval had higher rates of *perinatal* mortality. Eastman concluded, however, that the mother's age was more important than the birth interval, and that mothers should try to have their babies while still young, even if this meant close spacing of pregnancies. Statistical and computational techniques of the period did not permit satisfactory control for age and parity, or for social factors such as race and education of the mother.

Working about the same time, Yerushalmy[19] concluded that the birth interval was a significant factor in *perinatal* loss, and that longer intervals should be encouraged. However, in this study, the birth interval information was not available and age/parity categories were used as a proxy; it was assumed that a young mother of high parity must have had short birth intervals. Later work by Yerushalmy[20] using survey data found the same relationship (not controlling for age and parity) between interval and neonatal infant and child loss.

In a case-control study of all neonatal deaths in North Carolina, Spiers and Wang[13] matched cases on four variables (maternal age, race, education and parity) with controls who survived from all births in the state during 1969. A strong relationship was found between the length of the interpregnancy interval and *neonatal* death from a variety of causes, including sudden infant death syndrome. When birth weight was added as a fifth matching variable the relationship disappeared completely, leading the authors to conclude that birth interval influences neonatal mortality through the mechanism of birth weight.

Using data from the British Perinatal Mortality Survey of 1958, Fedrick and Adelstein[6] found that the optimum time between the termination of one pregnancy and the conception of the next appears to be between 6 and 12 months, and *perinatal* mortality for such infants is 15·1 per 1000 compared with 30·9 per 1000 for infants conceived in less than 6 months after the birth of their preceding sibling. After 12 months, however, the rate climbed very slowly to 30·5 deaths per 1000 births at 6 years (still lower than the rate after a very short interval), but climbed more steeply after that to 41·2 per 1000 at 9 years and 48·0 per 1000 for infants conceived more than 9 years after the previous infant. This work is particularly important for several reasons. First, it is based on national data (all births occurring in Britain during a single week, and all perinatal and neonatal deaths in the same area for a 3-month period, which included the same single week). Second, pregnancy interval rather than birth interval was used; if this is available it is preferable to use pregnancy interval. Infants born less than one year after their previous sibling include a disproportionate number of short gestation babies. A baby conceived 4 months after the termination of the previous pregnancy will be born less than a year after that termination if its gestation is 36 weeks or less, more than a year later if the gestation is 37 weeks or more, and its chances of survival are obviously much better if the gestation is longer. Thus the death rate of the short interval infants is spuriously increased when birth interval rather than pregnancy interval is used. Pregnancy interval data are often unavailable, however, especially in developing countries.

Finally, the Fedrick and Adelstein study is valuable because only pregnancy intervals following a surviving birth are analyzed. Only in this manner can the effect of the interval *per se* be separated from the effect of the outcome of the previous pregnancy. When another birth closely follows a stillbirth, it is not clear whether a poor outcome in the later birth can be attributed to the short interval or to the continuation of the detrimental factors that contributed to the poor outcome of the earlier birth.

In a study of nearly 100 000 pairs of siblings in Norway, Erikson and Bjerkedal[5] found that not only was the younger of the pair more likely to be low birth weight after a short birth interval, but the older of the pair was also more likely to be small at birth. Since the interval *after* the child's birth cannot possibly affect its birth weight, these authors concluded that the causal factor was not the birth interval *per se*.

Studies in developing countries have not examined *perinatal* mortality; they have, however, shown a relationship between birth interval and later mortality. Wyon and Gordon (1962)[18] working in the Punjab, Laurie and colleagues (1954)[7] in Kenya, Addo and Goody (1974)[1] in Ghana, and the World Health Organization in India, the Philippines, Iran, Turkey and Lebanon (Omran *et al.*, 1976)[9] all found a relationship between birth intervals and infant or early child mortality. None of these studies controlled maternal age and parity or the outcome of the previous pregnancy.

Wolfers and Scrimshaw (1975)[16], working in Ecuador, restricted analysis to infants whose predecessor survived and found that shorter birth intervals increased the probability of infant mortality in both the child who preceded the birth interval and the child who came after it.

It is clear that the relationship between birth interval and the outcome of pregnancy is a very complex one; there is a web of inter-relationships involving the age and parity of the mother, the outcome of the previous pregnancy or pregnancies and probably several social factors such as education.

The length of the interval between pregnancies is partly determined by the outcome of the earlier pregnancy. Unsuccessful pregnancies, i.e. those ending in miscarriage, stillbirth, neonatal or infant death, are followed more closely by another pregnancy than are those pregnancies ending in a live birth that continues to thrive[21]. Both physiologic and motivational factors are involved. A spontaneous abortion is followed by a shorter anovulatory period than a full-term pregnancy; a stillbirth is not followed by lactation that would have delayed the resumption of menstruation and ovulation; a neonatal or infant death prematurely terminates lactation and accelerates the concomitant return of ovulation; and finally, there is a tendency to 'replace' unsuccessful pregnancies[12].

Mother's age and parity are not independent of the pregnancy interval, and both of these are also related to the outcome of the pregnancy. Other things being equal, young mothers (< 18 years) and older mothers (> 30 years) have higher rates of perinatal mortality, and perinatal mortality increases after the second birth. A woman does not achieve high parity without either short birth intervals, advanced age or both. Is it the age or the parity or the short birth interval that has the greatest impact on the probability of the infant's survival? Do the three variables interact? Delayed childbearing is becoming increasingly common in some developed countries; is the older mother better off having her children close together, so that she will not be so old when her last child is born (as Eastman recommended 40 years ago), or is it more important to have the longer birth interval?

The outcome of the previous pregnancies also contributes to the parity level. Other things being equal, women with successful pregnancy outcomes are less likely to achieve the higher parities; they reach the same completed family size with fewer pregnancies than women with any kind of fetal or child loss. Whether each additional loss should be attributed to age, parity, birth interval or simply a continuation of conditions that produced the first loss is difficult to disentangle. The Norwegian study cited earlier suggests that the last explanation should not be discounted.

In this chapter we investigate the association between birth interval and two pregnancy outcomes: infant death and low birth weight. In addition to birth interval, maternal age and parity are treated as explanatory variables and the effect of previous pregnancy outcome is controlled by restricting the analysis to infants of women whose penultimate pregnancies ended in live offspring who remained alive at the time of the birth of the index child.

The data used for this analysis consist of 12 995 singleton births of second or higher order parity delivered in what was formerly called the Queen Farah Maternity Hospital in Tehran, Iran, in August 1977 and 1978. One of the largest maternity hospitals in the world, this hospital serves a population of primarily lower socio-economic status. Located in southern Tehran, it is one of several government hospitals in the city.

Two outcome variables are examined. The first is infant death occurring before the mother's discharge from the hospital ('perinatal mortality'); the death rate per 1000 deliveries is given. The second outcome variable is the incidence of births that weigh no more than 2500 g; the rate of low-birth-weight infants per 1000 deliveries is given.

The perinatal mortality measure just defined can be used to compare mortality in various subgroups within the study hospital. However, it should be used cautiously as a measure of comparison with other hospitals since postpartum hospitalization in the Queen Farah Maternity Hospital is short, less than 2 nights in 92% of the cases, and this clearly influences the level of reported mortality. This caveat applies to the discussion of mortality but not to discussion of birth weight.

Low birth weight is defined as ≤ 2500 g. We used this rather than the preferred < 2500 g[17] because of the tendency to round to the nearest whole number. However, this probably means that a certain proportion of the infants recorded as weighing exactly 2500 g are in fact slightly over 2500 g and are misclassified as being of low rather than normal birth weight. Only $3 \cdot 6\%$ of births are recorded as being 2500 g or less. Although this percentage is low, multiple births and first births are excluded, both of which would tend to raise the average birth weight. Since mothers whose previous pregnancy did not result in a live birth that is still living are also excluded, this, too, tends to raise the average birth weight, since a previous low birth weight infant is at the same time less likely to survive and to predict low birth weight in the index child.

For 557 of the 12 995 deliveries, there was no record of birth weight. However, we inferred from a comparison of the distributions of estimated gestational ages for babies with and without recorded birth weights that birth weights were similarly distributed in the two groups.

The two outcome variables are examined by categories of birth interval, parity and maternal age. Birth interval is categorized as 9–12,

13–24, 25–36, 37–48, 49–60, 61–72 and 73 or more months since the last pregnancy. This variable is treated as categorical rather than continuous because there is a strong tendency for women to report the number of months since the birth of their previous child with a number that is divisible by 12 (i.e. 12, 24, 36, etc.). At the longer birth intervals, there are probably an equal number of, say, 23 month and 25 month intervals reported as 24 months. However, in the shortest interval category (9–12 months), there are probably more reported as 12 months that should be 13 months than should be 11 months. This tendency would more likely produce an underestimate of the effect of the very short interval on birth weight. Although, as stated earlier, we would have preferred to use pregnancy, rather than birth interval, this was not available to us, and we did not think that the estimation of gestational age was reliable enough to calculate pregnancy interval.

Parity, including the index birth, is classified as 2 or 3, 4 or 5, and 6

Table 1   Some characteristics of women in different birth interval categories

| Characteristic | Interval since last birth (months) | | | | |
	≤ 12	13–24	25–36	> 37	Total
Number of cases	522	3844	3483	5146	12 995
Mean age	22·8	23·8	24·9	27·6	25·6
% with no education	75·2	73·8	74·8	71·6	73·3
% from urban area	95·1	93·8	92·9	92·8	93·3
% with any previous fetal or child loss	25·3	29·7	30·3	33·2	31·1
Mean number of surviving children	2·0	2·2	2·4	2·7	2·5
Mean number of pregnancies	2·5	2·8	2·9	3·3	3·0

or more. Maternal age in years is classified as less than 20, 20–29, and over 30.

The effects of the independent variables are estimated by using the linear logistic model[3]. Significance testing is accomplished by using asymptotic normal distribution theory. Risks of adverse outcomes at various levels of the explanatory variables are compared by estimating odds ratios.

Table 1 shows some of the characteristics of women in four interval categories. In terms of education and residence there is almost no difference by birth interval. However, women with longer birth intervals are older, as logically expected, and have had more reproductive events (pregnancies, living children and losses) consistent with their greater age.

Table 2 and Figure 1 clearly confirm the findings of previous researchers. As the interval between births lengthens, the *perinatal mortality* rates (before hospital discharge) decline sharply for the first 3

Table 2   Mortality before hospital discharge and incidence of infants with low birth weight ($\leq 2500\,\text{g}$) for different birth intervals

	Interval since last birth (months)							
	9–12	13–24	25–36	37–48	49–60	61–72	≥73	Total
Mortality								
No. of deliveries	522	3844	3483	1871	1240	779	1256	12 995
Deaths per 1000	34·5	22·6	14·6	16·0	22·6	18·0	27·9	20·2
Low birth weight								
No. of deliveries	503	3687	3331	1793	1177	747	1200	12 438*
LBW per 1000	99·4	40·4	31·8	29·0	28·9	20·1	34·2	35·9

* There are 557 cases with unknown birth weight

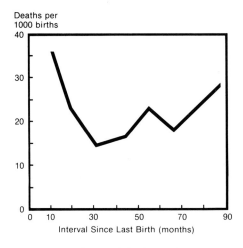

Figure 1   Infant mortality before hospital discharge by birth interval

years and then begin to increase. The mortality of infants born after a 2–4 year interval is less than half that of infants born after a very short interval (9–12 months). Although the decrease in mortality reverses after 3 years, it remains less at 6 years than it is in the 9–12 months interval.

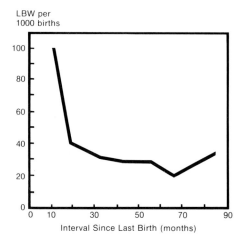

Figure 2   Incidence of low birth weight (LBW) (≤2500 g) by birth interval

As shown in Table 2 and Figure 2, the incidence of babies of *low birth weight* decreases steeply between 9 and 24 months since last birth. After 2 years, the incidence of low-birth-weight babies shows a slow downward trend until 6 years before it begins to increase again.

PARITY

Table 3 and Figure 3 show that the pattern between mortality and birth interval displayed in Figure 1 is maintained when the data are stratified by parity levels. Perinatal mortality rates decline for the first 2–3 years postpartum and then begin to increase. In general, mortality increases with parity; it is more than twice as high among women of parity 6 or higher (35 per 1000) as it is among women of parity 2 or 3 (14 per 1000). Based on the linear logistic model, there is no significant parity-interval interaction effect ($p>0\cdot10$) but both parity and interval contribute significant main effects ($p<0\cdot01$).

With regard to the interval effects, the largest risk of perinatal mortality is the shortest interval (9–12 months), and the odds ratios for perinatal mortality in the other intervals compared to the shortest are $1\cdot7$ for 13–24 months, $2\cdot6$ for 25–36 months and $2\cdot0$ for 37 or more months. When the parity effect is considered, the highest parity group (6+) has the greatest perinatal mortality, with the odds ratios for perinatal mortality in the remaining parity groups compared to the

Table 3   Mortality before hospital discharge and incidence of infants with low birth weight (≤2500 g) for different birth intervals, stratified by parity

| | *Interval since last birth (months)* | | | | |
Parity	9–12	13–24	25–36	≥ 37	Total
Mortality					
Parity 2 and 3					
No. of deliveries	349	2322	1944	2318	6933
Deaths per 1000	34·4	15·1	10·8	12·5	14·0
Parity 4 and 5					
No. of deliveries	121	922	1001	1848	3892
Deaths per 1000	24·8	20·6	20·0	26·5	23·4
Parity 6+					
No. of deliveries	52	600	538	980	2170
Deaths per 1000	57·7	55·0	18·6	29·6	34·6
Low birth weight					
Parity 2 and 3					
No. of deliveries	337	2230	1855	2226	6648
LBW per 1000	124·6	45·3	37·2	32·8	42·9
Parity 4 and 5					
No. of deliveries	116	886	957	1750	3709
LBW per 1000	34·5	32·7	23·0	22·9	25·6
Parity 6+					
No. of deliveries	50	571	519	941	2081
LBW per 1000	80·0	33·3	28·9	30·8	32·2

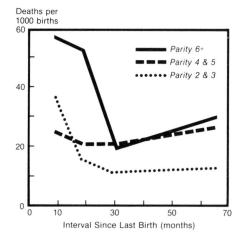

Figure 3   Infant mortality before discharge by birth interval, stratified by parity

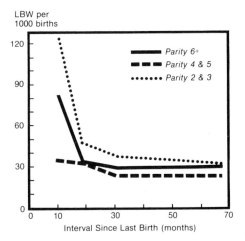

Figure 4 Incidence of low birth weight (LBW) (≤2500 g) by birth interval, stratified by parity

high parity group having values of 2·6 for parities 2 and 3, and 1·5 for parities 4 and 5. With the odds ratio estimates used for comparison, the effect of interval is about the same magnitude as the effect of parity.

In each parity stratum, the incidence of *low birth weight* declines over the first 2–3 years (Figure 4). The greatest interval effect is present in the low parity and high parity women where the incidence of low birth weight is more than 2·5 times higher for deliveries with a 9–12 month interval than for those with birth intervals of more than a year. Analysis by logistic regression indicates that there is no significant parity effect ($p > 0.50$) when comparing the high and low parity groups and that, overall, the main effects for interval are stronger than for parity, although both are significant ($p < 0.001$). Relative to the shortest interval (9–12 months), the odds ratio for low birth weight in the 13–24 months interval is 2·6 and is 3·2 and 3·5, respectively, for intervals of 25–36 and 37 or more months. The odds ratios for low birth weight in the parities 4 and 5 group and the parities 6 or larger group compared to the lowest parity group (2 and 3) are 1·6 and 1·3, respectively. By comparing the magnitudes of the odds ratios, it appears that the interval effects are uniformly stronger than the age effects.

AGE

For each stratum of maternal age shown in Table 4 and Figure 5, *perinatal mortality* decreases over the first 3 years of birth interval. When all maternal age–birth interval combinations are considered, babies of women younger than 20 years have the highest mortality (58 per 1000 deliveries) in the 9–12 month birth interval and the lowest mortality (8 per 1000 deliveries) for a birth interval greater than 3 years. However, if the 9–12 month birth interval is not considered, the perinatal mortality for babies of women younger than 20 does not differ significantly from that for the age group 20–29 years ($p > 0.05$). When the logistic regression model is used to estimate independent variables effects, both age and interval contribute significant main effects ($p < 0.001$).

The odds ratios associated with perinatal mortality for the birth

Table 4 Mortality before hospital discharge and incidence of infants with low birth weight ($\leq$ 2500 g) for different birth intervals, stratified by maternal age

	Interval since last birth (months)				
Age	*9-12*	*13-24*	*25-36*	*≥37*	*Total*
Mortality					
Age < 20 years					
No. of deliveries	137	642	345	121	1245
Deaths per 1000	58·4	12·5	11·6	8·3	17·9
Age 20-29 years					
No. of deliveries	308	2552	2388	3117	8365
Deaths per 1000	19·5	18·0	10·1	13·2	14·0
Age ≥ 30 years					
No. of deliveries	77	650	750	1908	3385
Deaths per 1000	51·9	50·8	30·7	34·1	36·9
Low birth weight					
Age < 20 years					
No. of deliveries	130	613	332	117	1192
LBW per 1000	153·8	52·2	51·2	68·4	64·6
Age 20-29 years					
No. of deliveries	229	2455	2286	2979	8019
LBW per 1000	76·9	38·3	31·1	23·5	32·2
Age ≥ 30 years					
No. of deliveries	74	619	713	1821	3227
LBW per 1000	94·6	37·2	25·2	35·1	34·7

(correction to page 122)

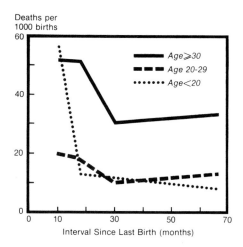

Figure 5   Infant mortality before hospital discharge by birth interval, stratified by age

intervals of 13–24 months, 23–36 months and 37+ months compared to the shortest interval (9–12 months) are, respectively, 1·6, 2·6 and 2·2. When the maternal age effect is considered, the oldest group (37 or more years) has the greatest overall perinatal mortality, with the odds ratios for perinatal mortality in the remaining age groups relative to the oldest group having values of 2·8 for ages 20–29 and 2·7 for ages <20. Through the use of odds ratios as an index for comparing effects, the interval and age effects are seen to be of the same order of magnitude.

The incidence of *low birth weight* declines in each age stratum through the 25–36 month birth interval (Table 4 and Figure 6). By the logistic regression model, both interval and age contribute significant main effects ($p<0·001$). For the interval effects, the greatest risk of giving birth to low-birth-weight infants is in the shortest interval (9–12 months), and the odds ratios for low birth weight in the other birth intervals when compared to the shortest are 2·5 for 13–24 months, 3·1 for 25–26 months and 3·3 for 37 or more months. With regard to the age effects, the risk of a low-birth-weight infant is highest in the youngest women (<20 years) and the odds ratios for low-birth-weight in the other age groups compared to the youngest women are 1·8 for women 20–29 years old and 1·5 for the women at least 30 years old. If the odds ratios are used as a basis of comparing the strengths of interval and age effects, the interval effects are uniformly stronger than those of age.

The interval between two births was examined for its effect on the proportion of the later infants who survive until their mothers are discharged from the hospital, and on the proportion of infants who weigh no more than 2500 g at birth. Maternal age and parity were controlled separately. Interval was found to be an important precursor of both perinatal mortality and low birth weight.

There are two important implications of these findings. First, it would appear that the older mother who wishes to have additional

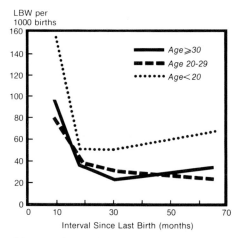

Figure 6   Incidence of low birth weight (LBW) (≤2500) by birth interval, stratified by age

children should be advised to wait until there is a satisfactory interval between the births, rather than to space the births closely in order to minimize her age at the later birth. A satisfactory interval is at least 2 years.

Second, all maternity hospitals should recognize the significance of the short birth interval to a high-risk pregnancy. Physicians delivering an infant born after a short interval should be aware of the increased probability of a low-birth-weight infant and take appropriate precautions.

Folk beliefs about the adverse effects of short birth spacing should be reinforced during postpartum contraceptive counseling, and appropriate contraceptive advice should be offered.

References

1 Addo, N. O. and Goody, J. (1974). *Siblings in Ghana.* Cambridge University and ISSER, University of Ghana, Legon
2 Caldwell, J. C. and Caldwell, P. (1977). The role of marital sexual abstinence in determining fertility: a study of the Yoruba in Nigeria. *Pop. Stud.,* **31**, 193
3 Cox, D. R. (1970). *The Analysis of Binary Data.* (London: Methuen)
4 Eastman, N. J. (1944). The effect of the interval between births on maternal and fetal outlook. *Am. J. Obstet. Gynecol.,* **47**, 445
5 Erikson, J. D. and Bjerkedal, T. (1979). Interval between pregnancies. Letter to the *Lancet,* 6 January, p. 52
6 Fedrick, J. and Adelstein, P. (1973). Influence of pregnancy spacing on outcome of pregnancy. *Br. Med. J.,* **4**, 753
7 Laurie, W., Brass, W. and Traut, H. (1954). *East African Medical Survey, Monograph 3 & 4.* (Nairobi: East African High Commission)
8 Morley, D. (1973). *Paediatric Priorities in the Developing World.* (London: Butterworths)
9 Omran, A. R., Standley, C. C., Azar, J. E. *et al.* (1976). *Family Formation Patterns and Health.* (Geneva: WHO)
10 Page, H. J. and Lesthaege, R. (eds.). (1981). *Child Spacing in Tropical Africa: Traditions and Change.* (New York: Academic Press)
11 Papavangelou, G. (1971). The Effects of Maternal Age, Parity and Concentration of Births on Selected Causes of Infant Mortality. *MSc dissertation,* London School of Hygiene and Tropical Medicine. (cited in reference 10)
12 Preston, S. H. (ed.). (1978). *The Effects of Infant and Child Mortality on Fertility.* (New York: Academic Press)
13 Spiers, P. S. and Wang, L. (1976). Short pregnancy interval, low birth weight and the sudden infant death syndrome. *Am. J. Epidemiol.,* **104**, 15
14 Ware, H. (1976). Motivation for the use of birth control: evidence from West Africa. *Demography,* **13**, 479
15 Williams, C. D. (1963). The story of kwashiorkor. *Courr. Cent. Int. Enf.,* **13**, 3661
16 Wolfers, D. and Scrimshaw, S. (1975). Child survival and intervals between pregnancies in Guayquil, Ecuador. *Pop. Stud.,* **29**, 479
17 World Health Organization (1980). *Statistics Quarterly,* **33**, 3
18 Wyon, J. B. and Gordon, J. E. (1962). A long-term prospective-type field study of population dynamics in the Punjab, India. In Kiser, C. V. (ed.). *Research in Family Planning.* (Princeton, NJ: Princeton University Press)
19 Yerushalmy, J. (1945). On the interval between successive births and its effect on the survival of the infant. *Hum. Biol.,* **17**, 65
20 Yerushalmy, J., Bierman, J. M., Kemp, D. H. *et al.* (1956). Longitudinal studies of pregnancy on the island of Kauai, Territory of Hawaii. 1. Analysis of previous reproductive history. *Am. J. Obstet. Gynecol.,* **71**, 80
21 Zimmer, B. (1979). Consequences of the number and spacing of pregnancies on outcome and of pregnancy outcome on spacing. *Soc. Biol.,* **26**, 161

Additional references

Gray, R. H. (1981). Birth intervals, postpartum sexual abstinence and child health. In Page, H. J. and Lesthaege, R. (eds.). *Child Spacing in Tropical Africa: Traditions and*

Change. (New York: Academic Press)
Wray, J. D. (1971). Population pressure on families: family size and child spacing. *Rep. Pop./Fam. Plann.*, Number 9

Section IV:
FAMILY PLANNING SERVICES IN THE MATERNITY HOSPITAL

10
Desire for additional children and contraceptive plans

D. J. NICHOLS and B. JANOWITZ

The Maternity Record contains but two attitudinal questions, appropriately placed at the very end of the interview schedule. Completed at the time of discharge from the hospital or maternity center, they record (1) the number of additional children desired by the individual and (2) plans for postpartum contraception. In evaluating the responses to these questions, it must be remembered that they reflect intentions and desires as they exist immediately following a pregnancy outcome. As such, they may be disproportionately influenced by the outcome of this pregnancy, as opposed to other factors which might be expected to be associated with future reproductive behavior.

In this chapter, we propose to examine the effect of child survival – including outcomes of previous pregnancies as well as the present one reported in detail on the Maternity Record – on the desire for additional children and plans for contraceptive use. Women who have had unsuccessful* pregnancy outcomes are more likely to want additional children and, consequently, will be less likely to plan to use contraception. In addition, unsuccessful past outcomes may encourage women to plan *additional* births as a form of 'insurance' against anticipated future infant or child mortality. In this way, mortality encourages women not only to *replace* non-surviving off-

---

* An unsuccessful pregnancy outcome is herein defined as a spontaneous abortion, stillbirth, or a non-surviving live birth. Because of the very different motivational factors associated with induced abortion, women reporting such outcomes for the previous pregnancy are excluded from this analysis.

spring, but also to plan for *extra* births because they expect that some number of living children will not survive, or that some proportion of future pregnancy outcomes will not result in a live birth.

If the replacement effect is an important factor in affecting the desire for additional children and the planned use of contraception, then women experiencing infant or child mortality will want to adjust for non-surviving offspring and, consequently, be less likely to use contraceptives. Full replacement would imply that women who have lost one child would want one more child than women who have lost none; women who have lost two, two more, and so on. The loss of the last child should have a larger impact on the desire for additional children than the loss of children of earlier birth orders. Subsequent pregnancies may have already replaced earlier child losses, while less time has been available for women to compensate for more recent losses, and none could yet have been made in response to the present outcome.

The impact of planning additional births to compensate for 'expected' child loss is difficult to measure. Since the Maternity Record collects information on the number of additional *children* desired but not explicitly on the number of additional *births* desired, it is therefore not possible to directly determine whether the latter exceeds the former. Some light, however, may be thrown on the importance of anticipated child loss as a factor influencing contraceptive plans. Women desiring the same number of additional children may be expected to have similar contraceptive plans. However, women who have had child losses may be more likely to expect losses in the future than women whose children have all survived. Such losses may cause women to delay contraception as they perceive the need to have more pregnancies than women who have not experienced child loss, even though they ultimately want the same number of surviving additional children.

THE DATA

For this analysis, we use records of 2110 deliveries occurring at Al Galaa Maternity Hospital, Cairo, between September 1977 and March 1979. Because the number and survival status of previous outcomes are of interest, we restrict the study population to women with two, three, or four total pregnancies* (including the current pregnancy) and examine each gravidity group separately (Table 1).

The average age of women completing their second pregnancy is slightly under 24 years. For women having a third delivery, the mean age is 26 years, and for those having a fourth outcome the mean age is nearly 28 years. One may infer from these data that childbearing in this study population begins after age 20, with roughly 2 year intervals between births. Approximately one half of the women in each gravidity group report one or more years of education.

The proportion reporting previous contraceptive use ('method mainly used before contraception', as it is referred to on the Maternity Record) increases from less than one fourth of the women completing a second pregnancy to 40% of those having a fourth outcome. What is *not* known, however, is the temporal relationship between interval contraceptive use and an ensuing pregnancy: did the woman discontinue use of a method *in order to* become pregnant, or was actual or perceived method failure the case?

The data on the survival status of the current pregnancy outcome indicate that, in this study population, second and third pregnancies

Table 1 Characteristics of women delivering at Al Galaa Maternity Hospital, Cairo (September 1977–March 1979)

	Total number of pregnancies including the current pregnancy		
	2	3	4
Mean age (years)	23·8	25·9	27·6
% Some education	53	50	49
% Previous contraceptive use	24	35	40
Previous outcomes			
% All surviving	67	50	41
% Last surviving	67	72	73
Mean no. living children	0·67	1·36	2·10
Current outcome			
% Surviving live birth	93	92	90
% Want more children	47	29	19
% Planned contraceptive use	68	77	82
Number of women	916	649	545

* 33% of all deliveries occurring during the reporting period (35% were first pregnancies, and 23% were fifth and higher order outcomes).

are slightly more likely to result in surviving neonates than fourth (and presumably higher-order) pregnancies. Additionally, the comparatively higher risk of *first* pregnancies is illustrated by the proportions surviving among the immediately *previous* pregnancy, when one compares that for gravidity two women (67%) with the corresponding proportions for gravidity three and four women (72–73%). The percentage of women whose previous pregnancy outcome was unsuccessful is very high in each of the three gravidity groups; at least one third of previous pregnancies had resulted in other than a surviving live birth by the time of the current delivery.

Earlier outcomes are similarly characterized by comparatively low survivorship. Among women with two previous pregnancies, only one half have two surviving children; among those with three previous pregnancies, the proportion with all surviving is as low as 41%.

As a consequence, the average number of living children at the time of the current delivery to women in each of the three gravidity groups is far below the number of pregnancies experienced: women with one previous pregnancy have an average of 0·67 children; those with two previous pregnancies, 1·36 survivors; and those with three previous pregnancies, 2·10 living children. We observe, however, that the *proportion* of surviving offspring (living children divided by pregnancies) is nearly equal in each of the three gravidity groups. Approximately 70% of all pregnancies – previous as well as current – have resulted in a surviving outcome.

Despite the high level of infant/child mortality, the desire to limit family size is fairly widespread, particularly among women with three or more pregnancies. Even among those with but one previous pregnancy – and including among them those with non-survivors – over one half do not wish to have additional children. These desires are reflected in the proportions intending to practice postpartum contraception: from 68% to 82% of the women in the three gravidity groups.

EFFECT OF PREVIOUS PREGNANCY OUTCOMES ON THE DESIRE FOR ADDITIONAL CHILDREN AND CONTRACEPTIVE PLANS

How do the results of previous pregnancy outcomes affect individual attitudes and intentions relating to future childbearing and contraception? To answer this question, we examine these relationships for women with one, two, and three pregnancies previous to the present outcome. The technique of analysis used is 'ordinary least squares regression using dummy variables', a procedure which enables the researcher to calculate the impact of a change in a single independent variable on the dependent variable, holding constant the effects of all other variables in the equation*.

Desire for additional children

Both the number and order of surviving outcomes affect the desire for additional children (Table 2). Among women with a surviving last outcome, the probability that a woman wants additional children decreases with an increase in the number of survivors. This result is found in all three gravidity groups; for example for women at gravidity 4 (including the present delivery), the probability that a woman wants additional children is 0·61 if she has one living child, 0·36 if she has two, 0·22 if she has three and 0·10 if all four children are alive. Similarly, if the woman's last outcome is not surviving, the probability of wanting additional children decreases with an increase in total number surviving. For the gravidity 4 group, the corresponding probabilities of wanting additional children are as follows: no living children, 0·73; one, 0·41; two, 0·20; and three, 0·08.

Controlling now for the *number* of surviving children, we found that women whose last child survived are more likely to report that they *do* want an additional child than are women whose last outcome did not survive; an exception is women at gravidity three with two surviving outcomes. It is not clear why the order of survivorship bears this relationship to the desire for additional children, as it is not consistent with the replacement hypothesis discussed above.

Before proceeding from these findings to a general conclusion that unsuccessful deliveries are causally linked to lower probabilities of desiring additional children, we must consider the temporal context of the administration of the Maternity Record to the individual woman.

---

* As described by Bowen and Finegan[1], the results of multiple regression may be described not only in terms of regression coefficients but also in terms of the adjusted rates or probabilities. Each adjusted rate may be interpreted as an estimate of an individual's being in category i of the dependent variable if she had otherwise been 'average' with respect to all other variables in the equation.

Table 2 Adjusted probabilities: desire for additional children (Al Galaa Maternity Hospital, Cairo: 1977–1979)*

Surviving children		Total number of pregnancies including the current pregnancy		
		2	3	4
None		0·89	0·72	0·73
One:	last surviving	0·72	0·60	0·61
One:	last not surviving	0·49	0·33	0·41
Two:	last surviving	0·32	0·17	0·36
Two:	last not surviving	—	0·25	0·20
Three:	last surviving	—	0·05	0·22
Three:	last not surviving	—	—	0·08
Four		—	—	0·10
Total		0·47	0·29	0·19
Number of women		916	649	545

* Other variables in the regression equation include the respondent's age, educational level, residence and proportion of previous pregnancies resulting in a living son

Questions are completed on the basis of information available at admission, during delivery and postpartum before the woman is discharged. It is quite possible that the outcome of the *current* delivery receives disproportionate weight (relative to previous outcomes) due to its 'immediacy' in the equation. While it cannot be tested with the data available, it may be that the postpartum euphoria following the birth of a healthy child – or the depression brought on by a stillbirth or neonatal death – is linked with immediate postpartum attitudes toward future childbearing.

Postpartum contraceptive plans

To the extent that family planning is practiced for the limitation of family size, a woman's planned contraceptive use will be dependent on whether she desires to have additional children. In the present investigation this variable is the most important in arriving at the adjusted probability of use in the open interval: at each gravidity shown in Table 3, approximately 90% of those who want no more children plan to use contraception, as do somewhat less than one half of those who do plan to have larger families.

Table 3 Adjusted probabilities: planned contraceptive use (Al Galaa Maternity Hospital, Cairo: 1977–1979)*

| | *Total number of pregnancies including the current pregnancy* | | |
	2	3	4
Previous outcomes			
None surviving	0·70	0·70	0·66
One surviving	0·63	0·73	0·74
Two surviving	—	0·81	0·87
Three surviving	—	—	0·83
Current outcome			
Not surviving	0·51	0·74	0·70
Surviving	0·69	0·78	0·84
Desire for addl. children			
No	0·88	0·91	0·90
Yes	0·46	0·41	0·44
Total	0·68	0·77	0·82
Number of women	916	649	545

* Other variables in the regression equation include the respondent's age, educational level, residence, proportion of previous pregnancies resulting in a living son and the proportion using contraception in the interval preceding the current delivery

Turning our attention to the respective outcomes of previous pregnancies and the current pregnancy, we found that the adjusted probability of planned contraception is positively associated with favorable outcomes, although differences net of the desire for additional children are small. Women who have had more successful outcomes tend to be more likely to plan to contracept than women who have had fewer successful outcomes.

Perhaps among women who want more children, those with a surviving last outcome are more motivated to delay the next pregnancy than are women with a non-surviving last outcome. Spacing considerations would then also be important, but less so than the desire to limit, in affecting postpartum contraceptive plans. It may also be that among limiters those with a surviving last outcome are more committed to the decision not to have another pregnancy.

Survival and contraceptive plans: an example

To assess the impact of improved survival on the desire for additional children and on contraceptive plans, we have calculated the appropriate proportions, within gravidity groups, under the assumption that infant and child mortality had existed at 75% of the reported level. For example, in Table 1 we read that, among gravidity two women, 67% of all *previous* outcomes and 93% of all *current* outcomes are surviving. Expressed in terms of mortality, 33% of previous pregnancies and 7% of current pregnancies are non-survivors. Applying a 25% reduction in these rates yields 25% not surviving among previous outcomes $(0 \cdot 33 \times 0 \cdot 75 = 0 \cdot 25)$, and 5% not surviving among current outcomes $(0 \cdot 07 \times 0 \cdot 75 = 0 \cdot 05)$.

Table 4 presents the results of this 'exercise'. Interestingly, it is only among women with *two* previous pregnancies (e.g. those having a third pregnancy outcome) that such a hypothetical mortality decline would have a substantial impact on the desire for additional children or the intention to practice family planning. For such women, the reduction would result in a drop by nearly one half (from 29% to 15%) in the proportion wanting more children, and an increase in the proportion planning to contracept from an already high 77% to 84%. For women with *one* or *three* previous pregnancies, as noted above, the effects of *aggregate* survival on the desire for additional children act in an opposite direction from that of survival *order* (see Table 2). Thus, while an increase in total survival *reduces* the desire for additional children, a reduction in the mortality associated with the last delivery tends to *increase* it. In such instances, a 25% improvement

Table 4 Desire for additional children and planned contraceptive use: as reported, and assuming a 25% reduction in mortality (Al Galaa Maternity Hospital, Cairo: 1977–1979)

Number of pregnancies*	Desire for additional children		Planned contraceptive use	
	Reported	25% Reduction	Reported	25% Reduction
2	0·47	0·43	0·68	0·70
3	0·29	0·15	0·77	0·84
4	0·19	0·19	0·82	0·82

* Including the current pregnancy

in survival results in only a negligible change in overall fertility and contraceptive plans. Furthermore, for women with *three* previous pregnancies, it is likely that the reported distributions are already skewed to such a degree that the reduction in mortality can add little to the balance: less than one of five women desires to have more children and over four of five intend to contracept.

Policy implications

We have illustrated, using data collected as part of the Maternity Care Monitoring program, that the survival status of previous pregnancy outcomes is an important determinant of both reproductive and contraceptive plans. Within gravidity groups, the number of favorable outcomes is inversely associated with the desire for additional children and directly associated with postpartum contraceptive plans. In addition, the desire for additional children is found to be the principal determinant of planned contraceptive use. An unanticipated, yet consistent, finding is that, within gravidity and survival categories, a higher probability of desiring additional offspring is associated with *favorable*, as opposed to unfavorable, current pregnancy outcomes: women who have just had a *surviving* live birth are more likely to want to have more children than are women who have just experienced unsuccessful pregnancy outcomes.

Furthermore, in examining the relative contributions of included variables on future contraceptive plans, we have shown that mortality continues to exert a measurable influence even when holding constant the desire for additional children. It is likely that both child spacing considerations and a measure of insurance against future child losses help to explain this relationship.

Viewed from a policy perspective, the findings of this study suggest that, particularly in developing societies with high levels of infant and childhood mortality and political-cultural barriers to the widespread acceptance of modern contraception, programs aimed at improving childhood survivorship are likely to have both direct and indirect effects on the use of family planning and fertility behavior. Despite the individual, family and societal benefits to be gained immediately as a consequence of improved survivorship, the present findings do not reveal a strong and consistent positive relationship between survivorship and contraceptive plans. Improved mortality appears to have no clear-cut impact on individual intentions to practice family planning as reported in the immediate postpartum period.

Reference

1 Bowen, A. and Finegan, O. (1969). *The Economics of Labor Force Participation*, p. 641. (Princeton, NJ: Princeton University Press).

11
Postpartum sterilization in São Paulo State, Brazil

B. JANOWITZ, J. LEWIS, D. COVINGTON and M. S. NAKAMURA

Female sterilization is the second most popular contraceptive method in the state of São Paulo, Brazil. At the time of a contraceptive prevalence survey in 1978, 63·9% of all currently married women aged 15–44 were using contraception; of these, 25% had been sterilized[3]. Access to sterilization is limited by knowledge of where to obtain the service, and this knowledge is positively correlated with education, although education does not affect interest in sterilization[1].

Although a 1942 law prohibits Brazilian physicians and hospitals from providing information on any treatment that prevents pregnancy or interrupts gestation, the Medical Code of Ethics states that sterilization can be performed under exceptional circumstances after consultation with, and approval by, two physicians[4]. Legal barriers to sterilization have proved less important in practice than on paper. As with access to other modern methods of family planning – pills, IUDs and condoms – access to sterilization may be limited more by inability to arrange and pay for services than by legal restrictions.

This chapter describes and analyzes factors affecting planned and actual sterilizations among women in hospitals for obstetric deliveries, at five hospitals in the city of Campinas, São Paulo State. Wherever possible, the data from maternity patients are compared with survey data.

While this analysis relates to hospitals in Campinas, hospital records from Rio de Janeiro show similar patterns of sterilization among obstetric patients in that city, indicating that the problems of access described here may be generalized to other parts of the country.

São Paulo is the most developed state in Brazil; it has the highest per capita income, a good highway system and a well-developed communications network[3]. It is an area characterized by declining fertility rates. Like the rest of Brazil, the population of the state of São Paulo is overwhelmingly Roman Catholic and is becoming increasingly urban[2]. Campinas, a city of approximately 600 000 inhabitants, is estimated to have the highest per capita income in the state of São Paulo.

Data on 10 692 women having obstetric deliveries were collected from January 1977 to April 1979 at five hospitals in Campinas. Except for the number of beds, there is little difference in the facilities or services available at each of the five hospitals. There is also little difference in the characteristics of the maternity patients at each hospital.

In this analysis, in testing for association between any two variables, the statistic "tau c" is used throughout. All relationships that are significant are at the 1% level.

STERILIZATION PLANS AND IMPLEMENTATION

Effects of education and parity

All women were asked how many additional children they wanted. For this analysis, women who want no more children constitute the group who might consider postpartum sterilization as a method of family planning.

Of all the women, 40% wanted no more children (Table 1) and desire for additional children decreased as the woman's level of education increased. This, however, is because the women with less education are of higher parity, and not because education itself is associated with future pregnancy intentions. When parity is controlled, there are few systematic differences in the desire for additional children associated with education, for at any given parity, women within the higher education groups are generally no more likely than women with less education to say they want no more children. For parities of two or more, there is no significant association between education and the desire for no more children. Only a very small proportion of women with one child wanted no more children. Indeed, among those with one

Table 1 Percentage of currently married women aged 15–44 who want no more children, by parity and education: Campinas Maternity Record data

| Parity | Education (years) | | | Total |
	<3	3–4	>4	
1	17·6 (165)*	6·2 (1372)	3·7 (1901)	5·4 (3438)
2	56·3 (199)	40·0 (1120)	47·9 (745)	44·4 (2064)
3	82·6 (138)	87·5 (626)	86·4 (301)	86·6 (1065)
≥4	96·0 (272)	95·4 (560)	94·4 (125)	95·4 (957)
Total†	69·5 (863)	44·4 (3813)	26·6 (3122)	40·1 (7798)

* Numbers of cases in parentheses
† Including women with 0 or unknown parity

child, education is negatively correlated with the percentage of women desiring no more children and this relationship is significant.

Among maternity patients who wanted no more children, 42% indicated that they planned to be sterilized. There is no significant association between education and sterilization plans (Table 2). By comparison, data obtained from the statewide survey[3] indicated that 44·4% of women who had all the children they wanted were interested in being sterilized.

Over 60% of maternity patients planning to be sterilized are actually sterilized. Education has a pronounced effect on whether the

Table 2 Sterilization plans and follow-through for currently married women aged 15–44, by education level: Campinas Maternity Record data

| | Education (years) | | | Total |
	<3	3–4	>4	
% of maternity patients who want no more children:				
Planning sterilization	43·9 (574)*	40·8 (1655)	43·3 (818)	42·0 (3047)
Actually sterilized	18·3	24·7	30·8	25·1
% of maternity patients planning sterilization who were actually sterilized	43·4 (251)	62·0 (673)	72·3 (354)	61·2 (1278)

* Numbers of cases in parentheses; women with unknown contraceptive plans are excluded

sterilization takes place. Only 43·4% of women with 3 or fewer years of education were sterilized prior to leaving the hospital, compared with 72·3% among women with secondary schooling. Thus, among women who have all the children they want, plans for sterilization are not affected by education, but the percentage of women actually sterilized increases with education. While the percentage of women sterilized is less than that predicted from Nakamura's[3] survey population, the positive correlation is in agreement with that predicted by the survey.

Table 3 Average parities for currently married women by age and sterilization status: Campinas Maternity Record data and state of São Paulo Contraceptive Prevalence Survey (Nakamura et al., 1980)[3]

| | Average parity | | |
| | Campinas women planning sterilization* | | São Paulo survey women sterilized postpartum |
Age (years)	Actually sterilized	Not sterilized	
20–24	3·07 (101)†	3·42 (33)	2·56 (21)‡
25–29	3·49 (267)	4·12 (141)	3·73 (76)
30–34	3·76 (226)	4·80 (192)	4·08 (59)
35–39	4·29 (126)	6·19 (81)	4·82 (31)
40–44	5·48 (42)	7·23 (22)	§ (9)
Total	3·76 (762)	4·85 (469)	4·07 (196)

* Including all women who reported that they wanted no more children
† Numbers of cases in parentheses
‡ Unweighted numbers
§ Not calculated if $n < 20$

Average parity is higher among women who did not obtain sterilization than among women who did. Since women with the higher levels of education are more likely to be sterilized and since average parity is negatively correlated with education, it is not surprising that the women actually sterilized are of lower average parity, 3·76, than those not sterilized, 4·85, (Table 3). A t-test indicates that these differences are significant except for the age group 20–24.

The average parity of maternity patients receiving sterilizations compared with that of women in Nakamura's survey who were sterilized postpartum is higher, 4·07 to 3·76, but differences are small.

Effect of age and parity

As expected, the percentage of women wanting no more children is positively correlated with age (Table 4). Only one quarter of the women aged 20–24 want no more children compared with almost all women aged 40–44. Older women are, of course, likely to be of higher parity than younger women; and controlling for parity reduces, but does not eliminate, the generally positive and significant association between the desire for no more children and age. As women age, caring for a newborn is less acceptable and less appealing.

Table 5 shows that, as expected, among women who do not want any more children the percentage planning to be sterilized increases significantly with age. Younger women who do not want additional children are less likely to be interested in a permanent method of contraception. Therefore, some young women who say they want no more children may mean 'in the foreseeable future' but are not yet ready to take such a final step.

Among those planning sterilization, however, there is an unexpected negative and significant correlation between education and the percentage of women sterilized. Since younger women have had more years of education than older women, this negative correlation may reflect the negative relationship between education and the achievement of sterilization plans in this age group.

There is a positive and significant correlation between age and the percentage of women sterilized among those wanting no more children. Therefore, among all women eligible for sterilization, i.e. those wanting no more children, the positive correlation between plans and age outweighs the negative correlation between actualization and age, so that, overall, there is a positive correlation between sterilization and age.

Access to sterilization

Whether a woman carries out her plans to be sterilized depends, in part, upon her ability to work within the organizational constraints of the Brazilian medical care structure, to arrange and pay for surgery. There are, basically, three mechanisms of payment in Brazil, (1) private patients pay their own fees, (2) non-private patients are not charged for care and (3) insured patients pay their costs by social or

Table 4 Percentage of currently married women aged 15–44 wanting no more children, by age and parity: Campinas Maternity Record data

Parity	Age (years)					
	15–19	20–24	25–29	30–34	35–39	40–44
1	7·0 (795)*	4·7 (1598)	3·2 (817)	10·0 (190)	22·2 (36)	† (2)
2	48·3 (205)	40·7 (838)	41·4 (707)	51·6 (252)	80·0 (60)	† (9)
3	† (19)	79·3 (328)	87·9 (428)	92·3 (221)	98·2 (57)	† (13)
≥4	† (3)	89·0 (136)	95·0 (321)	96·0 (299)	100·0 (145)	100·0 (46)
Total‡	16·6 (1022)	27·8 (2969)	44·7 (2338)	67·5 (1002)	87·4 (340)	98·0 (102)

* Numbers of cases in parentheses
† Not calculated if $n < 20$

Table 5 Sterilization plans and follow-through for currently married women aged 15–44, by age: Campinas Maternity Record data

	Age (years)					
	15–19	20–24	25–29	30–34	35–39	40–44
% of maternity patients who want no more children:						
Planning sterilization	1·9 (160)*	17·2 (801)	42·0 (1016)	63·7 (672)	72·6 (292)	67·3 (98)
Actually sterilized	0·6	12·6	26·5	33·9	42·9	42·0
% of maternity patients planning sterilization actually sterilized	† (3)	75·4 (138)	64·8 (426)	53·5 (428)	60·0 (210)	63·6 (66)

* Numbers of cases in parentheses; women with unknown contraceptive plans are excluded
† Not calculated if $n < 20$

private insurance. 'Insured' is a residual category composed of all women who said they were neither private nor public patients. The reasonableness of the assumption that they are insured patients can be tested by comparing the distribution of patient status for all obstetric patients at one hospital with published information supplied by the hospital for 1978 (Table 6).

Table 6   Comparison of Maternity Record and hospital data on patient status

Status	Maternity record data %	Published hospital data %
Private	5·1	7·4
Insurance	82·5	83·1
Non-private or free	12·4	9·5

Table 7 shows that private patients are the most likely to be sterilized (87%), followed by insured patients (61%) and non-private patients (39%). These differences are significant at the 1% level.

Payment status is affected by education. Of women with fewer than 3 years of education, less than 1% were private patients, but of women with at least 5 years of education, 22·9% were private patients. The percentage of non-private patients decreases with education: 2 years or less of education, 14%; 3-4 years, 8%; and 5 or more years, 6%. The

Table 7   Percentage of women sterilized among women who want no more children and plan to be sterilized, by patient status and education

Patient status	Education (years)							
	<3		3-4		>4		Total	
	No.*	%	No.	%	No.	%	No.	%
Private	0	†	6	†	81	89	87	87
Insured	215	45	616	64	252	70	1083	61
Not private	36	36	51	41	20	40	107	39
Total	251	43	673	62	353	72	1277	61

* Numbers of cases on which percentages are based
† Not calculated if $n < 20$

percentage of women whose care is paid for by insurance is not affected by education.

Interaction between education and payment status does not affect the probability that a woman obtains sterilization. Taken together, education and payment status explain a slight but significant amount of the variance in the percentage of women who are sterilized ($R^2 = 0 \cdot 06$) with each factor accounting for about half the variance explained. Both financial factors and knowledge of how to make arrangements for surgery are important influences on obtaining sterilization. The role of these two factors requires further study.

Following a pattern that seems to be characteristic for Brazil, the rate of cesarean sections at these hospitals is extremely high. More than 40% of all deliveries were by this method, compared with 10–15% at most hospitals in the United States and western Europe. Analysis of recorded medical data on these deliveries indicates that in the Brazilian hospitals a substantial proportion are elective sections at this delivery, or the result of cesarean delivery of a previous pregnancy.

The data from these hospitals show that most women who were sterilized had cesarean deliveries. Of 783 women who are sterilized, 758 (97%) also had cesarean sections. This percentage is markedly higher than in other countries. For example, data from the United States for 1975 indicate that of all sterilizations performed at the time of delivery, only 27% were concurrent with a cesarean section. The probability that a woman who is sterilized also had a cesarean section varies little by education or payment status. Women who are not sterilized have a much lower rate of cesarean deliveries, but sterilizations at delivery are rarely carried out for women with vaginal deliveries. Apparently, a major justification for the high cesarean rate is that they are performed to provide sterilizations.

For women who want no more children, cesarean deliveries appear to be an unnecessarily expensive way to obtain sterilizations. One estimate for Brazil indicated that the difference in price between a cesarean and a vaginal delivery at a private clinic is US $1500 (US $2500 versus US $1000). If we assume that this same differential prevails for all deliveries in Campinas, then the additional charge for performing sterilizations concurrently with cesarean sections for all 758 of the sterilized women who had delivered their babies vaginally and were sterilized postpartum may be as high as US $1 137 000 ($758 \times \$1500$).

While women having vaginal deliveries have a shorter hospital stay than women having abdominal deliveries, the addition of sterilization would be expected to extend the time in hospital for women delivered vaginally more than for women with cesarean deliveries, and this would tend to reduce further the cost differential. The data for Campinas, however, indicate that, when sterilization is added to delivery, the additional nights required in hospital are about equal for the two types of delivery and do not affect the cost differential.

An interesting question is the extent to which variations in hospital policies may influence whether or not a woman is sterilized. Hospital policies may influence a woman to become interested in sterilization and, if she is interested, affect whether she is actually sterilized. To test for a hospital effect, the women were divided into three groups based on the hospital where the birth took place.

The percentage of women wanting no more children varies by hospital (Table 8), but these differences may be explained by variations in the average number of living children for obstetric patients at the three hospitals. Although the proportion of women reporting that they want no more children is highest at hospital C, so is average family size. The proportion of women reporting that they want no more children is lowest at hospital A, and so is average family size.

Among women who want no more children, there are large variations by hospital in the proportions who plan to be sterilized (Table 8). The highest proportion is among those delivering at hospital A and the lowest is at hospital C. Two factors may influence this

Table 8   Selected characteristics related to sterilization among women with obstetric deliveries in three hospitals in the Campinas area

	Hospital		
	A	B	C
% of women who want no more children	47·5 (4998)	49·6 (561)	57·0 (242)
% planning sterilization	47·9 (2313)	26·9 (275)	12·4 (137)
% actually sterilized*	30·1 (2313)	12·4 (275)	10·2 (137)
% of sterilized women who had cesarean sections	98·1 (697)	82·4 (34)	† (14)
% of unsterilized women who had cesarean sections	4·2 (409)	10·3 (39)	† (3)

* Base is women who want no more children
† Not calculated if $n < 20$

difference: (1) whether hospital policies and staff actively promote family planning, including sterilization, through such mechanisms as counseling and education programs, and (2) whether women select hospitals according to their policies on family planning and sterilization. The data available on characteristics of the women provide no insights about why women go to a particular hospital. There may be other factors for which data were not collected that predispose women to deliver in one hospital rather than another. Additional data need to be collected to determine the influence of hospital policies, staff attitudes and practices and women's preferences on their plans for sterilization. If, as these data strongly suggest, sterilization is available only in conjunction with a cesarean delivery, more information is needed on how women actually go about planning and making the necessary arrangements for a postpartum sterilization.

Sixty-one percent of the women in this study who planned sterilization were actually sterilized postpartum, virtually all of the sterilizations being in conjunction with a cesarean delivery. While cesarean sections accounted for an extremely high percentage of deliveries at these hospitals, this type of delivery – and concurrent sterilization – is not equally available to all women who indicated a desire to be sterilized. Whether a woman is actually sterilized is strongly correlated with her level of education and her payment status, suggesting that her knowledge of how to make the necessary arrangements and her ability to pay for services are determining factors. This has the effect of limiting access for those women most in need of sterilization, since poor women with low levels of education are also of highest parity.

Providing sterilization only in conjunction with cesarean delivery is costly, and restricts even further its availability to women who cannot pay for services, either from their own funds or from third-party coverage. These costs could be reduced substantially by making sterilizations available with vaginal deliveries.

References

1 Janowitz, B., Anderson, J. E., Morris, L., Nakamura, M. S. and Fonseca, J. B. (1980). Service availability and the unmet need for contraceptive and sterilization services in São Paulo State, Brazil. *Int. Fam. Plann. Perspect.*, 6
2 Moreira, M., da Silva, L. and McLaughlin, R. (1978). *Brazil. Country Profiles.* (New York: Population Council)

3 Nakamura, M. S., Morris, L., Janowitz, B., Anderson, J. E. and Fonseca, J. B. (1980). Contraceptive use and fertility levels in São Paulo State, Brazil. *Stud. Fam. Plann.*, **11**
4 Rodrigues, W., de Proenca, J. A. G., Paiva, M. A., Mattoso, R. DeQ., de Affonseca, L., de Paiva, Q. A., Nogueina, T. and Filho, B. M. (1975). Law and Population in Brazil. *Law and Population Monographs Series* No. 34. (Medford, Massachusetts: Tufts University)

12

Access to sterilization in two hospitals in Honduras

B. JANOWITZ and J. NUNEZ

Female sterilization is one of the most widely used family planning methods in Latin America. For example, data from recent contraceptive prevalence surveys indicate that 16% of the currently married women 15–44 years of age in the State of São Paulo, Brazil, have been sterilized[3]. The comparable figure for El Salvador is 18%[2] and for Panama, 30%[1]. (The Panama data are for women 20–49 years of age.)

Little is known about contraceptive use in Honduras because no contraceptive prevalence survey has been done there. Data collected from women having obstetric deliveries at hospitals in the major cities of Tegucigalpa and San Pedro Sula have provided information about these women's past contraceptive use and plans for postpartum contraception. This chapter focuses upon these women's plans for postpartum sterilization and factors that affect whether those plans are carried out.

Data for this analysis were collected at the Hospital Materno–Infantil in Tegucigalpa and the Hospital Leonardo Martinez in San Pedro Sula. The Hospital Materno–Infantil is the country's major maternity hospital. It is a large, well-equipped, university-affiliated hospital that serves the capital city's population as well as patients referred from the surrounding rural areas. The Hospital Leonardo Martinez in San Pedro Sula is a general hospital that serves as the major primary care and referral center for the coastal area. This region is more economically depressed than that served by the Hospital Materno–Infantil.

Analysis of these data indicates that the hospitals do not encourage women to be sterilized, and also that they do a poor job of providing services for those who are interested in sterilization.

Of 18 523 women giving birth from 1977 through 1979, 13 241 (71·5%) indicated that they did not want any more children. These women thus constituted a group for which female sterilization could be the contraceptive method of choice.

Of these 13 241 women, 3063 (23·2%) said they planned to be sterilized. In general, women who make this statement have large families. Almost 85% have four or more living children, and over 25% have seven or more children. Of the women who said they planned to be sterilized, only one tenth were actually sterilized postpartum.

Little variation was found between the two hospitals providing sterilization services with regard to preferred practices or the age and education of the patients. Though personnel at both hospitals preferred to do sterilizations 6–7 weeks after delivery, there is reason to believe that many women did not return to the hospital for surgery.

Among women having abortions at these hospitals, about half do not return for a follow-up visit 4–6 weeks later. (The two hospitals' records for the period 1977–1978 indicate that 56·7% of the women return for abortion follow-up in Tegucigalpa and 41·4% return in San Pedro Sula.) If follow-up is equally poor for obstetric patients desiring sterilization, then the practice of not performing the surgery at the time of delivery stops many women from obtaining sterilization.

To be eligible for sterilization in Honduras, one is supposed to satisfy the 'rule of 80' (living children times age must equal 80). It might be thought, therefore, that many women were not sterilized because they failed to meet this criterion. However, as Table 1 shows, 27·7% of the women who were sterilized at the two hospitals did not satisfy this rule.

In contrast, the data in Table 2 indicate that only 6·8% of the women who planned to be but were not sterilized, did not satisfy this rule. If the requirement of meeting the rule were the determining factor affecting who is actually sterilized, then it would be expected that the percentage of women not meeting the 'rule of 80' would be lower among sterilized women than among those not sterilized. Since the data indicate that the relationship is exactly the opposite, it must be that other factors are more important in determining who gets sterilized.

An alternative hypothesis is that scarce operating room time is the most important factor affecting who obtains a sterilization. If that were the case, women admitted to the operating room for purposes other than sterilization (e.g. obstetric complications) should find it easier to obtain a sterilization than other women. That is because the former group would have medical reasons other than sterilization for finding a place in an already-crowded operating room schedule, whereas obstetric patients with no medical complications would find it more difficult to have surgery scheduled.

One way to test this hypothesis is to consider the women planning sterilization and to compare those with different types of deliveries in terms of the percentage sterilized. If the hypothesis is valid, women with cesarean deliveries should have a higher probability of being sterilized than women with vaginal deliveries.

At both hospitals, the percentages of women delivered by cesarean section were low compared to the percentages so delivered at hospitals in other countries. In the United States, for example, between 15 and 20% of all deliveries are abdominal. In developing countries, where the majority of uncomplicated births occur at home, and a disproportionate share of hospital deliveries involve complications, one might expect the rate of cesarean deliveries to be at least as high. However, of all deliveries studied at the two Honduran hospitals, only 6·4% of those at Tegucigalpa and 2·8% of those at San Pedro Sula were abdominal deliveries.

Among the women who were sterilized, however, the percentage of those who had cesarean deliveries was a surprising 69% – 67% at Tegucigalpa and 73% at San Pedro Sula (see Table 1). In contrast, of the women who said they planned to be sterilized but were not sterilized at delivery, less than 1% had cesarean sections (Table 2). Therefore, it seems apparent that women who have abdominal deliveries find it easier to obtain a sterilization at the time of delivery than do women with vaginal deliveries.*

It may be argued that among women planning sterilization, those with cesarean deliveries were more likely to satisfy the 'rule of 80' than women with vaginal deliveries. This difference could then partly explain the higher rate of sterilization among women with abdominal deliveries.

* Over 99% of the women who were sterilized and had cesarean sections had made their plans before delivery. Patients undergoing emergency cesareans do not get sterilized because the necessary paperwork has not been done (personal communication from hospital staff).

Table 1 Sterilized women with cesarean and vaginal deliveries, showing the percentage not satisfying the 'rule of 80'

Hospital location	Type of delivery					Total		
	Vaginal		Cesarean					
	No. sterilized	% not satisfying 'rule of 80'	No. sterilized	% not satisfying 'rule of 80'	No. sterilized	% not satisfying 'rule of 80'	Percentage of deliveries that were cesareans	
Tegucigalpa	67	17·9	136	35·3	203	29·6	67·0	
San Pedro Sula	27	7·4	73	30·1	100	24·0	73·0	
Total	94	14·9	209	33·5	303	27·7	69·0	

Table 2 Women desiring sterilization who were not sterilized, by type of delivery, showing the percentages not satisfying the 'rule of 80'[a]

Hospital location	Type of delivery					Total		
	Vaginal		Cesarean					
	No. of women	% not satisfying 'rule of 80'	No. of women	% not satisfying 'rule of 80'	No. of women	% not satisfying 'rule of 80'	Percentage of deliveries that were cesareans	
Tegucigalpa	1841	6·0	11	b	1852	6·4	0·6	
San Pedro Sula	650	7·7	9	b	659	8·2	1·4	
Total	2491	6·4	20	b	2511	6·8	0·8	

[a] A total of 249 women whose age, parity, or method of delivery was unknown have been excluded from these data
[b] Numbers too small to permit meaningful analysis of proportions not satisfying the 'rule of 80'

At both hospitals, however, the proportion of sterilized women who did not satisfy the rule was higher among those with cesarean deliveries than among those with vaginal deliveries. For example, at the Hospital Materno–Infantil, 35·3% of the sterilized women studied who had cesareans failed to satisfy the rule, as compared to 17·9% of those who had vaginal deliveries. Women with cesarean deliveries thus appear less likely to satisfy the legal requirements for sterilization than do women with vaginal deliveries. Furthermore, among women with vaginal deliveries, the percentage not satisfying the 'rule of 80' was higher among those sterilized (14·9%) than among those not sterilized (6·4%).*

It may still be argued that women sterilized concurrently with cesarean delivery have a cesarean section at least in part to simplify procedures required to obtain a sterilization. For all women who were sterilized, however, the data indicate that in nearly all cases where a cesarean section was performed there was ample justification for the procedure. In fact, there are good arguments to support doing more cesarean sections among the group with vaginal deliveries. For example, the usual medical practice would be to perform an abdominal delivery for any woman who previously had a cesarean section; yet, of the 109 women sterilized at the time of delivery, eight with previous cesarean sections were delivered vaginally.

The data also indicate that many women delivered vaginally who planned to be sterilized but were not had strong indications favoring cesarean section. That is, of the 2673 women with vaginal deliveries, 58 previously had cesareans and 1135 (42·5%) had some other condition that would be considered an indication for cesarean section.

This chapter focuses on two findings – the very low rate of post-partum sterilization at two hospitals in Honduras and the high proportion of sterilizations that are done concurrently with cesarean sections. These two findings may be explained by one set of circumstances.

Both hospitals are crowded, and operating room time is scarce. Women who are already in the operating room because they are having cesarean sections can be sterilized using only a small amount of additional operating room time. Other women who want to be

* As may be seen in Table 2, the number of women who had cesarean sections and desired sterilization but were not sterilized was too small to permit meaningful comparison of the proportion not satisfying the 'rule of 80', vis-a-vis the proportion that had cesarean sections and were sterilized but did not satisfy the rule.

sterilized are likely to be sterilized only if an operating room happens to be free when they deliver their babies.

These circumstances also help to explain why the 'rule of 80' is more often broken for women with cesarean sections than for those with vaginal deliveries. The former group have medical reasons for cesarean sections, which may indicate that future pregnancies would be difficult; over 40% of the women sterilized at the time of a cesarean section, for example, had previously had a cesarean section. Therefore, given such stronger contra-indications for future pregnancies, it was to be expected that the group with cesarean sections should be less likely to meet the formula requirements for sterilization – as was in fact the case. In addition, much of the regulatory paperwork involved in performing a sterilization is reduced if the procedure can be justified on medical grounds. We may therefore conclude that a major factor restricting sterilizations at both hospitals has been available space, particularly operating room space.

The limitation on operating room space may also explain why personnel at these hospitals preferred to do interval rather than post-partum sterilizations. Interval sterilizations can be fitted into a busy operating room schedule at some specific time (for example, the Hospital Materno–Infantil does six interval laparoscopic sterilizations every Tuesday). Postpartum sterilization not concurrent with cesarean sections can rarely be done, since operating room time is not likely to be available.

At present, two operating rooms for sterilization at the Hospital Materno–Infantil have been equipped but are not yet operational. It is expected that with this increase in facilities, the demand for sterilization at this hospital can be more adequately met. Plans are currently underway for evaluating the impact of these new facilities.

References

1 Mascarin, F., Anderson, J. E. and Monteith, R. S. (1979). *Final Report, 1981. Family Planning Maternal and Child Health Survey*. Republic of Panama
2 Morris, L., de Mendoza, A. M., Anderson, J. E., Warren, C. W. and Rugamas, R. C. (1979). The use of contraceptive prevalence surveys to evaluate the family planning program in El Salvador. Presented at the *Annual Meeting of the American Public Health Association*, November 4–8, New York, USA
3 Nakamura, M. S., Morris, L., Janowitz, B., Anderson, J. E. and Fonseca, J. B. (1980). Contraceptive use and fertility levels in São Paulo State, Brazil. *Stud. Fam. Plann.*, **11**, July–August

Index

157